£12.50

PATHWAYS THROUGH SURGICAL FINALS

For Churchill Livingstone

Publisher: Laurence Hunter
Project Editor: Dilys Jones
Copy Editor: Sukie Hunter
Indexer: Nina Boyd
Production Controller: Lesley Small
Sales Promotion Executive: Marion Pollock

PATHWAYS THROUGH SURGICAL FINALS

J. A. Britto BSc MBBS

SHO in Neurosurgery, Royal London Hospital, London, UK
Currently Resident in General Surgery, Beth Israel Hospital, Boston, USA

M. J. R. Dalrymple-Hay BSc MBBS

SHO in Orthopaedics, Royal National Orthopaedic Hospital, London, UK

CHURCHILL LIVINGSTONE
EDINBURGH LONDON MADRID MELBOURNE NEW YORK AND TOKYO 1993

CHURCHILL LIVINGSTONE
Medical Division of Longman Group UK Limited

Distributed in the United States of America by Churchill Livingstone
Inc., 650 Avenue of the Americas, New York, NY 10011, and by
associated companies, branches and representatives throughout the
world.

First published 1993

ISBN 0-443-04806-1

British Library Cataloguing in Publication Data
A catalogue record for this book is available from the British Library.

Library of Congress Cataloging in Publication Data
A catalog record for this book is available from the Library of
Congress.

The
publisher's
policy is to use
**paper manufactured
from sustainable forests**

Produced by Longman Singapore Publishers (Pte) Ltd.
Printed in Singapore

CONTENTS

PREFACE

HOW TO USE THIS BOOK

In presenting the reader with these pathways, we hope to encourage a method of learning which is based on problem-solving. You will already have a general knowledge of the essential disciplines of pathology and the spectrum of clinical presentation of disease. We would expect anyone hoping to make best use of this text to have already a working knowledge of basic clinical medicine and surgery and to be able to examine patients confidently at the bedside. This book aims to give you an appreciation of differential diagnosis and put the facts into perspective. We emphasise the importance of directed history-taking, examination and choice of investigations on the route to diagnosis. Brief notes on treatment are included, either at the end of the pathway with the diagnosis or, where certain principles need emphasizing, in a separate section.

This book is *not* designed for rote learning in order to pass exams, because by its nature it cannot contain every fact about the conditions herein. It is, however, designed to promote a method of thinking that will make clinical decision-making on the wards, and in clinic and casualty, interesting and rewarding. It will also enable you to plan essay answers for surgical final examinations that will convince your examiners that you are safe and able to take a wide view when presented with clinical problems.

Best use of the pathways themselves might be made by covering the page and attempting to predict the major discriminating decisions as the pathways develop. We have been consistent in the use of capitals, bold type and font and in the use of boxes for diagnoses. We do not wish to prejudice the reader down any particular path, but it must be emphasized that prevalence is an important feature in diagnosis, and the safe clinician always considers the treatable, common condition early in the differential diagnosis. Thus the most common diagnoses feature in bold in a shaded box, less common diagnoses bold in an unshaded box and rarer conditions in normal type in an unshaded box. As an 'aide memoire' we have included 'rarer differential diagnoses' – do not ignore these!

We have included case histories for a few presenting complaints. After working through the book, the reader should be able to answer the questions posed and form a management plan based on the differential diagnosis. The case histories will thus provide a useful self-test facility.

The routes to diagnosis are not absolute, and different teachers may feel that certain clinical features and/ or discriminating investigations bear different emphases. We do not claim a monopoly on the diagnostic art! However, we hope to have provided a starting point, a framework of theory, which the reader may later care to modify by experience.

Best of luck!

ACKNOWLEDGEMENTS

The development of this text from a simple idea to the completed collection of pathways was made possible by Mr William Woods DM, FRCS, Consultant General Surgeon, Worthing Hospital, who has reviewed and edited all the relevant material. We are very grateful for the many hours of discussion and comment that he contributed and acknowledge the great amount that we were able to learn in the writing and editing process.

We would also like to acknowledge the help and advice of the following surgeons who contributed advice and editorial comment:

Mr Mike Dilkes FRCS	Ear, nose and throat
Mr Steven Bryan FRCS, FCOphth	Ophthalmology
Mr Bryan Jenkins MD, FRCS	Urology
Mr Gareth Scott FRCS	Orthopaedics

Boston and London 1993

J.A.B.
M.J.R.D.-H.

SECTION A

GENERAL SURGERY

ABDOMINAL PAIN

INTRODUCTION

This subject is covered in Chapters 1 and 2.

The aim of these chapters is to emphasise the major features which separate life-threatening conditions from those which demand less immediate action. The major discriminant clinical features and their significance are shown, and the appropriate investigations indicated.

Almost any condition may reflect as abdominal pain, whether the offending organ is abdominal or not. The diagnosis is particularly difficult when the patient is a child or elderly person, and when the clinical picture is indistinct. Conditions which may provoke the symptom include myocardial infarction, lobar pneumonia, diabetic ketoacidosis, sickle cell disease and a variety of other rarer differential diagnoses outside the scope of this text.

Case history

A 40-year-old vagrant who is a regular attender at the local A & E department is brought into hospital with acute abdominal pain of 2 hours duration. He is a known alcoholic with previous admissions for head injuries and haematemesis. The patient is lying flat, unwilling to move and crying out in pain. The pain is constant, unremitting and severe and the patient has vomited twice with no haematemesis. There are no symptoms referrable to the urinary tract.

On examination the patient is normotensive, in sinus rhythm 90 per minute and apyrexial. He has a tense rigid abdomen, with tenderness on palpation and release. There are no bowel sounds and no organomegaly, distension or ascites. Rectal examination is normal.

1. What is the immediate differential diagnosis and what does the doctor do next?

The diagnosis of generalized peritonitis is made, due to pancreatitis or perforated duodenal ulcer. The patient is kept 'nil by mouth', and an intravenous fluid regime is started.

2. What is the major discriminant investigation, and what other investigations are important and why?

The casualty officer notes a mildly raised amylase and thereby excludes a diagnosis of pancreatitis. Normal FBC, WBC, liver function and glucose are noted. Blood gases are normal and an erect CXR reveals subdiaphragmatic gas.

3. What is the diagnosis and how is the patient further managed?

An urgent surgical referral is made and the duty surgical registrar arranges urgent laparotomy, at which a large perforated duodenal ulcer is oversewn.

1. THE ACUTE ABDOMEN

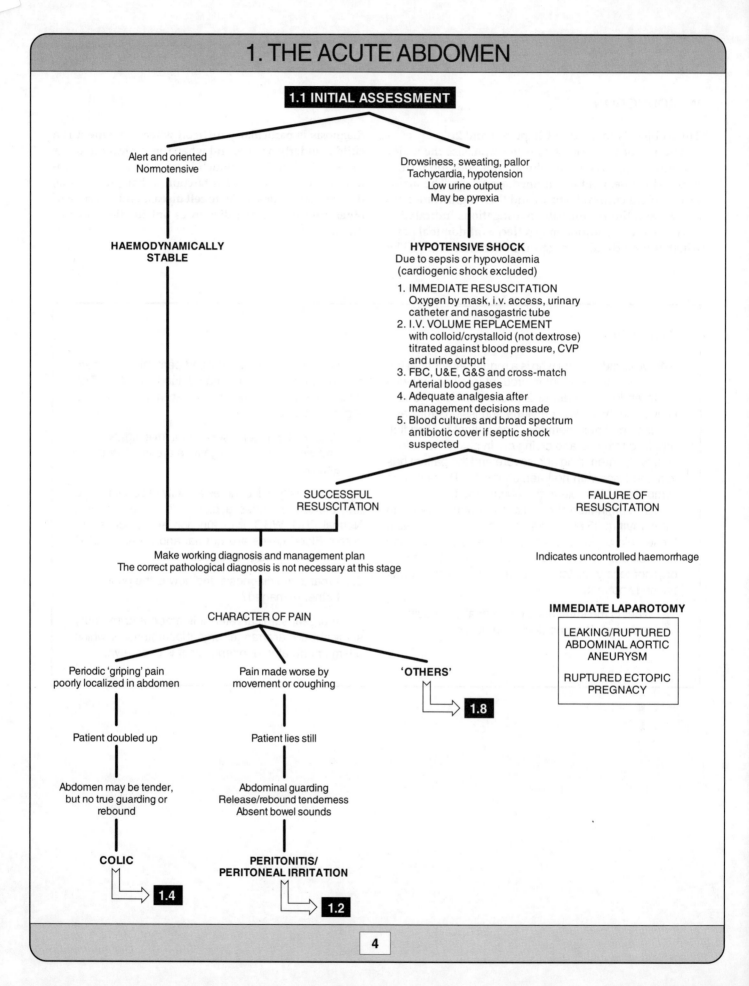

1.1 INITIAL ASSESSMENT

**Alert and oriented
Normotensive**

**HAEMODYNAMICALLY
STABLE**

**Drowsiness, sweating, pallor
Tachycardia, hypotension
Low urine output
May be pyrexia**

HYPOTENSIVE SHOCK
Due to sepsis or hypovolaemia
(cardiogenic shock excluded)

1. IMMEDIATE RESUSCITATION
   Oxygen by mask, i.v. access, urinary
   catheter and nasogastric tube
2. I.V. VOLUME REPLACEMENT
   with colloid/crystalloid (not dextrose)
   titrated against blood pressure, CVP
   and urine output
3. FBC, U&E, G&S and cross-match
   Arterial blood gases
4. Adequate analgesia after
   management decisions made
5. Blood cultures and broad spectrum
   antibiotic cover if septic shock
   suspected

SUCCESSFUL
RESUSCITATION

FAILURE OF
RESUSCITATION

Make working diagnosis and management plan
The correct pathological diagnosis is not necessary at this stage

Indicates uncontrolled haemorrhage

IMMEDIATE LAPAROTOMY

LEAKING/RUPTURED
ABDOMINAL AORTIC
ANEURYSM

RUPTURED ECTOPIC
PREGNACY

CHARACTER OF PAIN

Periodic 'griping' pain
poorly localized in abdomen

Pain made worse by
movement or coughing

'OTHERS'

1.8

Patient doubled up

Patient lies still

Abdomen may be tender,
but no true guarding or
rebound

Abdominal guarding
Release/rebound tenderness
Absent bowel sounds

COLIC

1.4

**PERITONITIS/
PERITONEAL IRRITATION**

1.2

1. THE ACUTE ABDOMEN

1.2 PERITONITIS

GENERALIZED PERITONITIS
Continued resuscitation

LOCALIZED PERITONITIS
→ 1.3

'Nil by mouth', intravenous fluids
(May pass nasograstric tube)

SERUM AMYLASE PLUS ERECT CHEST X-RAY

Normal or slightly raised amylase
May be free gas on X-ray,
best seen under the diaphragm

Greatly raised amylase
No free gas on X-ray,

Suggests:

PERFORATED VISCUS

LAPAROTOMY

Causes include:

Suggests:

ACUTE PANCREATITIS

Management aims:

1. Continued resuscitation
2. Support cardiac, respiratory and renal function
   Maintain electrolyte balance and nutrition - this may involve inotropes, ventilation and parenteral fluids, electrolytes and feeding regimens
3. Establish cause in the stable patient

ULTRASOUND SCAN

GALLSTONE

No evidence of gallstone

Majority of cases

Other common causes

Rarer causes

Crohn's ileitis
Perforated Meckel's diverticulum

Perforation in:
-Duodenal ulcer
-Gastic ulcer
-Gastric carcinoma
-Colonic diverticulum
-Colonic tumour
-Inflamed appendix

Mesenteric infarction

Perforation in:
-Strangulated, obstructed small bowel
-Sigmoid volvulus
-Caecal volvulus
-Gallbladder

Ruptured:
-Ovarian cyst
-Ectopic pregnancy
-Tubal abscess

Majority of cases

Rarer differential diagnosis

Toxic drugs
Infective (mumps)
Pancreas divisum

Idiopathic
Alcoholic

4. Operation usually for complications, (CT scan is investigation of choice)
   - pseudocyst, abscess, necrosis

1. THE ACUTE ABDOMEN

1.3 LOCALIZED PERITONITIS

Gynaecological symptoms predominate
Consider clinical evidence for gynaecological
sepsis and investigate appropriately

Gastrointestinal symptoms predominate
Nausea, vomiting, 'flatulent dyspepsia'
Diarrhoea, constipation

Right upper quadrant pain
referred to shoulder tip,
worse on inspiration

Central abdominal pain
moving to the right iliac fossa

Left iliac fossa pain

May be tender local mass

May be tender local mass

May be tender local mass

Right-sided tenderness
on rectal examination

Left-sided tenderness
on rectal examination

ULTRASOUND
Thickened gallbladder wall;
may be gallstones

Routine blood tests and
plain X-rays unhelpful

Routine blood tests and
plain X-rays unhelpful

ACUTE CHOLECYSTITIS

'Nil by mouth'
Intravenous fluids
Antibiotics
(May pass nasogastric tube)

**ACUTE APPENDICITIS
SUSPECTED**

ACUTE DIVERTICULITIS

'Nil by mouth'
Intravenous fluids
Antibiotics
(May pass nasogastric tube)

Resolution

Failure to resolve or deterioration
(consider acalculous cholecystitis
in the ITU patient after burns,
sepsis, trauma)

Urgent
cholecystectomy

Cholecystectomy
either first available
list or 6 weeks later

Resolution

Failure to resolve
or deterioration
suggests perforation
or abscess formation

Laparotomy

Appendicectomy

By open incision
or laparoscopy

Clinical picture complicated
by gynaecological
symptoms –
LAPAROSCOPY

Inflamed appendix
Septic fluid

Normal appendix

Likely causes:
– Perforated peptic ulcer
– Mesenteric adenitis
– Perforated caecal carcinoma
– Crohn's disease

Gynaecological causes

Likely causes:
– Tubo-ovarian sepsis
– Ruptured ectopic pregnancy
– Ruptured ovarian cyst

ACUTE APPENDICITIS

1. THE ACUTE ABDOMEN

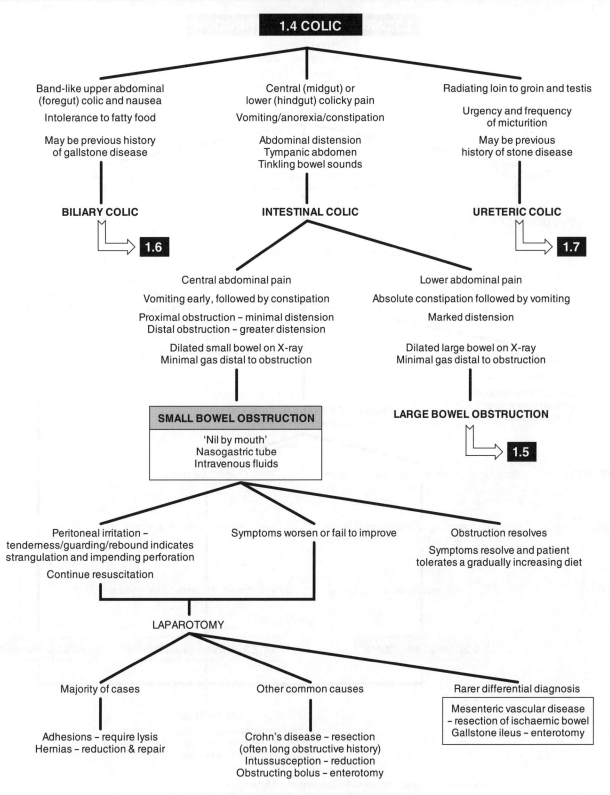

1.4 COLIC

Band-like upper abdominal (foregut) colic and nausea

Intolerance to fatty food

May be previous history of gallstone disease

BILIARY COLIC → **1.6**

Central (midgut) or lower (hindgut) colicky pain

Vomiting/anorexia/constipation

Abdominal distension
Tympanic abdomen
Tinkling bowel sounds

INTESTINAL COLIC

Radiating loin to groin and testis

Urgency and frequency of micturition

May be previous history of stone disease

URETERIC COLIC → **1.7**

Central abdominal pain

Vomiting early, followed by constipation

Proximal obstruction – minimal distension
Distal obstruction – greater distension

Dilated small bowel on X-ray
Minimal gas distal to obstruction

SMALL BOWEL OBSTRUCTION
'Nil by mouth'
Nasogastric tube
Intravenous fluids

Lower abdominal pain

Absolute constipation followed by vomiting

Marked distension

Dilated large bowel on X-ray
Minimal gas distal to obstruction

LARGE BOWEL OBSTRUCTION → **1.5**

Peritoneal irritation – tenderness/guarding/rebound indicates strangulation and impending perforation

Continue resuscitation

Symptoms worsen or fail to improve

Obstruction resolves

Symptoms resolve and patient tolerates a gradually increasing diet

LAPAROTOMY

Majority of cases

Adhesions – require lysis
Hernias – reduction & repair

Other common causes

Crohn's disease – resection
(often long obstructive history)
Intussusception – reduction
Obstructing bolus – enterotomy

Rarer differential diagnosis

Mesenteric vascular disease
– resection of ischaemic bowel
Gallstone ileus – enterotomy

In all cases the aims of laparotomy are to 1. Decompress dilated bowel
2. Reduce/release the obstruction
3. Resect ischaemic bowel and allow primary anastomosis

1. THE ACUTE ABDOMEN

1.5 LARGE BOWEL OBSTRUCTION

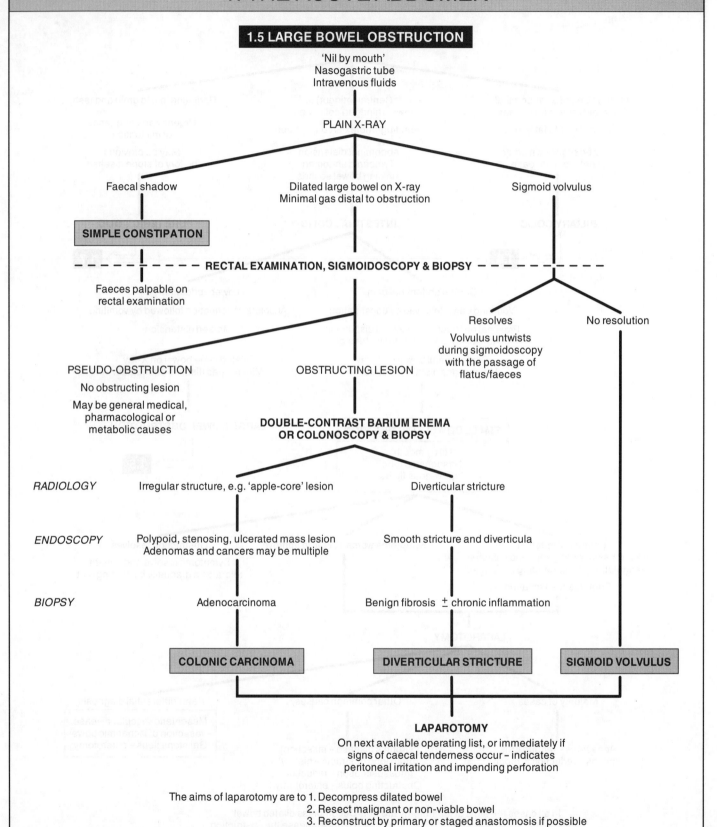

'Nil by mouth'
Nasogastric tube
Intravenous fluids

PLAIN X-RAY

Faecal shadow

Dilated large bowel on X-ray
Minimal gas distal to obstruction

Sigmoid volvulus

SIMPLE CONSTIPATION

RECTAL EXAMINATION, SIGMOIDOSCOPY & BIOPSY

Faeces palpable on
rectal examination

Resolves

Volvulus untwists
during sigmoidoscopy
with the passage of
flatus/faeces

No resolution

PSEUDO-OBSTRUCTION

No obstructing lesion

May be general medical,
pharmacological or
metabolic causes

OBSTRUCTING LESION

**DOUBLE-CONTRAST BARIUM ENEMA
OR COLONOSCOPY & BIOPSY**

RADIOLOGY   Irregular structure, e.g. 'apple-core' lesion   Diverticular stricture

ENDOSCOPY   Polypoid, stenosing, ulcerated mass lesion   Smooth stricture and diverticula
Adenomas and cancers may be multiple

BIOPSY   Adenocarcinoma   Benign fibrosis ± chronic inflammation

COLONIC CARCINOMA   **DIVERTICULAR STRICTURE**   **SIGMOID VOLVULUS**

LAPAROTOMY

On next available operating list, or immediately if
signs of caecal tenderness occur – indicates
peritoneal irritation and impending perforation

The aims of laparotomy are to 1. Decompress dilated bowel
2. Resect malignant or non-viable bowel
3. Reconstruct by primary or staged anastomosis if possible

1.6 BILIARY COLIC

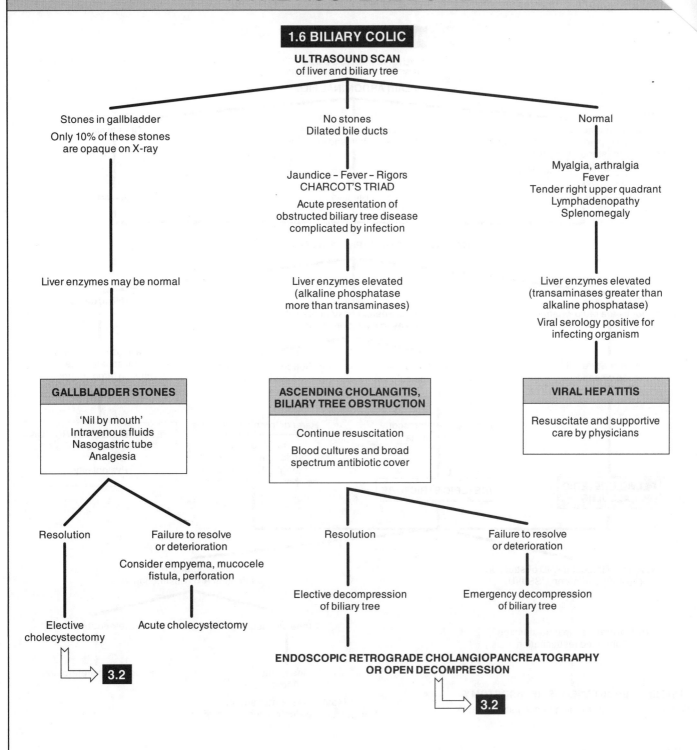

ULTRASOUND SCAN
of liver and biliary tree

Stones in gallbladder

Only 10% of these stones
are opaque on X-ray

Liver enzymes may be normal

GALLBLADDER STONES

'Nil by mouth'
Intravenous fluids
Nasogastric tube
Analgesia

Resolution

Failure to resolve
or deterioration

Consider empyema, mucocele
fistula, perforation

Elective
cholecystectomy

Acute cholecystectomy

3.2

No stones
Dilated bile ducts

Jaundice – Fever – Rigors
CHARCOT'S TRIAD

Acute presentation of
obstructed biliary tree disease
complicated by infection

Liver enzymes elevated
(alkaline phosphatase
more than transaminases)

**ASCENDING CHOLANGITIS,
BILIARY TREE OBSTRUCTION**

Continue resuscitation

Blood cultures and broad
spectrum antibiotic cover

Resolution

Failure to resolve
or deterioration

Elective decompression
of biliary tree

Emergency decompression
of biliary tree

**ENDOSCOPIC RETROGRADE CHOLANGIOPANCREATOGRAPHY
OR OPEN DECOMPRESSION**

3.2

Normal

Myalgia, arthralgia
Fever
Tender right upper quadrant
Lymphadenopathy
Splenomegaly

Liver enzymes elevated
(transaminases greater than
alkaline phosphatase)

Viral serology positive for
infecting organism

VIRAL HEPATITIS

Resuscitate and supportive
care by physicians

1.7 URETERIC COLIC

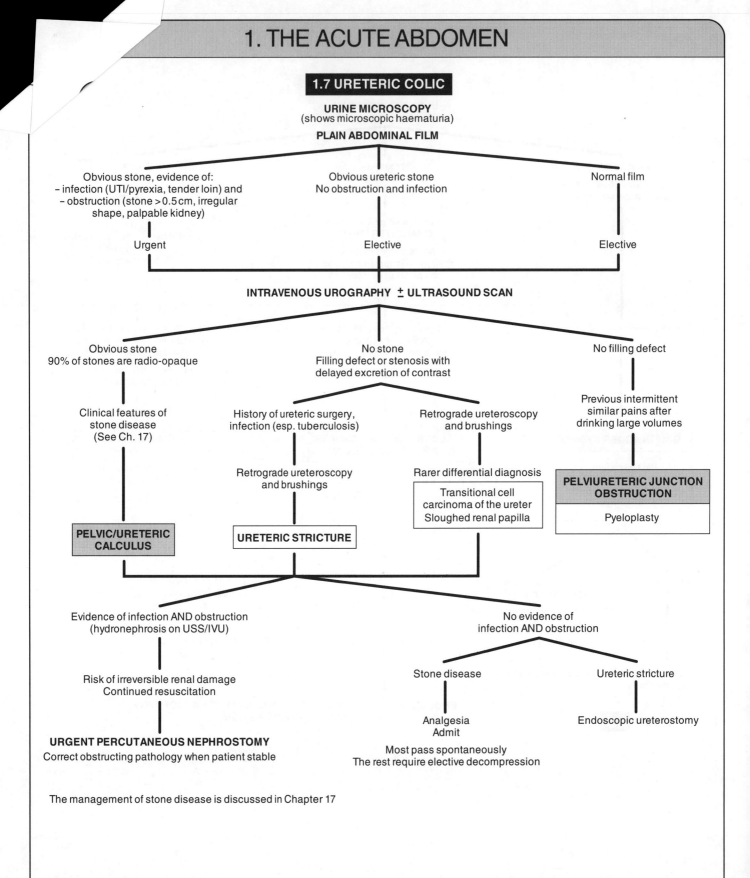

URINE MICROSCOPY
(shows microscopic haematuria)

PLAIN ABDOMINAL FILM

Obvious stone, evidence of:
– infection (UTI/pyrexia, tender loin) and
– obstruction (stone > 0.5 cm, irregular
shape, palpable kidney)

Obvious ureteric stone
No obstruction and infection

Normal film

Urgent

Elective

Elective

INTRAVENOUS UROGRAPHY ± ULTRASOUND SCAN

Obvious stone
90% of stones are radio-opaque

No stone
Filling defect or stenosis with
delayed excretion of contrast

No filling defect

Clinical features of
stone disease
(See Ch. 17)

History of ureteric surgery,
infection (esp. tuberculosis)

Retrograde ureteroscopy
and brushings

Previous intermittent
similar pains after
drinking large volumes

Retrograde ureteroscopy
and brushings

Rarer differential diagnosis

Transitional cell
carcinoma of the ureter
Sloughed renal papilla

**PELVIURETERIC JUNCTION
OBSTRUCTION**

Pyeloplasty

**PELVIC/URETERIC
CALCULUS**

URETERIC STRICTURE

Evidence of infection AND obstruction
(hydronephrosis on USS/IVU)

No evidence of
infection AND obstruction

Risk of irreversible renal damage
Continued resuscitation

Stone disease

Ureteric stricture

Analgesia
Admit

Endoscopic ureterostomy

URGENT PERCUTANEOUS NEPHROSTOMY
Correct obstructing pathology when patient stable

Most pass spontaneously
The rest require elective decompression

The management of stone disease is discussed in Chapter 17

1. THE ACUTE ABDOMEN

1.8 'OTHERS'

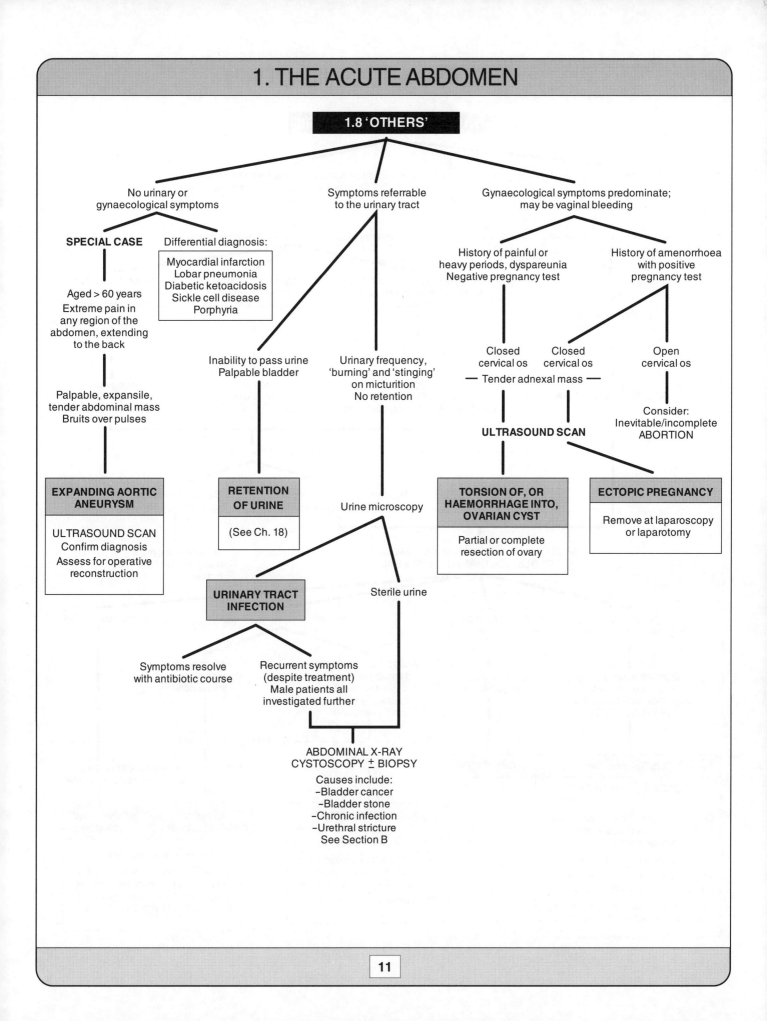

No urinary or gynaecological symptoms

SPECIAL CASE

Aged > 60 years
Extreme pain in any region of the abdomen, extending to the back

Palpable, expansile, tender abdominal mass
Bruits over pulses

EXPANDING AORTIC ANEURYSM

ULTRASOUND SCAN
Confirm diagnosis
Assess for operative reconstruction

Differential diagnosis:

Myocardial infarction
Lobar pneumonia
Diabetic ketoacidosis
Sickle cell disease
Porphyria

Symptoms referrable to the urinary tract

Inability to pass urine
Palpable bladder

RETENTION OF URINE

(See Ch. 18)

Urinary frequency, 'burning' and 'stinging' on micturition
No retention

Urine microscopy

URINARY TRACT INFECTION

Sterile urine

Symptoms resolve with antibiotic course

Recurrent symptoms (despite treatment)
Male patients all investigated further

ABDOMINAL X-RAY
CYSTOSCOPY ± BIOPSY

Causes include:
–Bladder cancer
–Bladder stone
–Chronic infection
–Urethral stricture
See Section B

Gynaecological symptoms predominate; may be vaginal bleeding

History of painful or heavy periods, dyspareunia
Negative pregnancy test

History of amenorrhoea with positive pregnancy test

Closed cervical os

Closed cervical os
— Tender adnexal mass —

Open cervical os

Consider:
Inevitable/incomplete ABORTION

ULTRASOUND SCAN

TORSION OF, OR HAEMORRHAGE INTO, OVARIAN CYST

Partial or complete resection of ovary

ECTOPIC PREGNANCY

Remove at laparoscopy or laparotomy

2. CHRONIC ABDOMINAL PAIN

2.1 UPPER ABDOMINAL PAIN

Unremitting, severe epigastric pain

Episodic symptoms which may be severe: relieved by antacids/H_2-blockers

History of NSAID or alcohol abuse and smoking

History of smoking, NSAID or alcohol abuse

Cachexia and weight loss
Anaemia

Palpable Virchow node
and malignant liver
May be epigastric mass

Retrosternal pain/discomfort
worse on bending, lying down
– 'heartburn'

Postprandial epigastric
pain/discomfort
dissuades from eating

Preprandial upper
abdominal pain,
relieved by milk/antacids

Suggests:
GASTRIC CARCINOMA

Suggests:
OESOPHAGITIS/
OESOPHAGEAL ULCERATION

Suggests:
BENIGN
GASTRIC ULCER

Suggests:
BENIGN
DUODENAL ULCER

Trial of antacids, FBC & MCV

No improvement of symptoms
Iron deficiency anaemia

Symptoms improve
Haematology normal

**UPPER GASTROINTESTINAL ENDOSCOPY
± DOUBLE-CONTRAST BARIUM MEAL**

MILD 'DYSPEPSIA'
Usually resolves without
further investigation

Oesophageal
ulceration/inflammation

Widespread superficial
gastric inflammation

Discrete deep stomach ulcer

Duodenal ulceration

Stomach may herniate
via the diaphragm
into chest with acid reflux:
HIATUS HERNIA

Petechial
haemorrhage

Rolled, heaped edge
Loss of elasticity
in rigid stomach
Usually not
on lesser curve

Smooth edge
Most commonly
on lesser curve

– – – – – – – – – – – – – – BIOPSY (multiple sites) – – – – – – – –

Adenocarcinoma

Benign inflammation and may reveal
infective cause, e.g. *Helicobacter pylori*

OESOPHAGITIS/
OESOPHAGEAL ULCER
Columnar adenomatous metaplasia =Barrett's oesophagus (may be premalignant)
Conservative treatment
– lose weight, stop smoking, alcohol – antacids, H_2-blockers, omeprazole
For persistent symptoms and failure of medical treatment – operation

GASTRITIS

GASTRIC CARCINOMA
No metastases – resect for cure
Metastatic disease – operation for palliation of symptoms (e.g. pain/bleeding/obstruction)
Chemotherapy may be of use

BENIGN GASTRIC ULCER	DUODENAL ULCER
Conservative treatment	
–lose weight, stop smoking, alcohol –antacids, H_2-blockers, omeprazole –metronidazole and amoxycillin for presumptive *H. pylori* infections	

2. CHRONIC ABDOMINAL PAIN

2.2 EXACERBATION OF COLICKY PAINS

Exacerbation of small-bowel colicky pains, especially after meals
Nausea and vomiting, distension/bloating

Exacerbation of large-bowel colicky pains

May be combination of:
– urgency and frequency at stool,
– diarrhoea – constipation – mucus/pus per rectum

SIGMOIDOSCOPY & BIOPSY
(Flexible sigmoidoscopy reaches splenic flexure)

Normal

Polypoid, stenosing or ulcerated mass lesion
Polyps may be multiple

Inflammation and mucosal bleeding

May be constipated bowel loaded with faeces

(Defer biopsy if barium enema to be performed within 2 weeks because of risk of perforation)

COLITIS

BARIUM MEAL & FOLLOW-THROUGH/ SMALL-BOWEL ENEMA

DOUBLE-CONTRAST BARIUM ENEMA ± COLONSCOPY & BIOPSY

RADIOLOGY

Normal

Stricture, deep 'rose-thorn' ulcers, 'cobblestones', ± fistulae in segmental 'skip' distribution

Mucosal ulcers and granularity
Pseudopolyps
Dilatation

Obligate rectoproximal distribution

Diverticular strictures

Normal colon loaded with faeces

ENDOSCOPY & BIOPSY
(Crosby capsule in small-bowel disease)

Normal

Inflammation in discontinuous 'skip' lesions
Deep ulcers
'Cobblestones'

Continuous inflammation
Pseudopolyps
Dilatation

Chronic inflammation and diverticula

Normal colon loaded with faeces

Granulomatous full-thickness disease

Non-granulomatous mucosal disease

Chronic inflammation only

IRRITABLE BOWEL SYNDROME	CROHN'S ILEITIS	CROHN'S COLITIS	ULCERATIVE COLITIS	DIVERTICULAR DISEASE	CONSTIPATION
Symptomatic treatment Reassurance		(See p. 41)		Antibiotics and supportive care in the acute phase	Purgatives

INTRODUCTION

Jaundice is the yellow pigmentation of skin or sclera caused by hyperbilirubinaemia. It manifests itself when the serum bilirubin exceeds 60 µmol/l.

The causes of jaundice are:

a. Overproduction of bilirubin related to intravascular or extravascular haemolysis (prehepatic)
b. Impaired liver uptake, conjugation or secretion of bilirubin (hepatic)
c. Obstruction to the outflow of bile (posthepatic)

Case history

A 72-year-old man presents to his general practitioner with a history of 8 weeks of pruritus and 5 weeks of progressive painless jaundice. Further questioning reveals that he has had clay-coloured stools and dark urine for 5 weeks. He has been otherwise well.

1. What features in this history are suggestive of obstructive jaundice?

2. What feature favours a malignant cause?

General examination reveals yellow sclerae. The gallbladder is palpable. Biochemical analysis reveals a pattern of obstructed jaundice.

3. What products of bilirubin metabolism would you expect to be:
   a. present in the urine?
   b. absent from the urine?

4. What relative values of transaminases and alkaline phosphatase will be found in the serum?

Ultrasound shows a dilated biliary tree with an irregular lesion in the head of the pancreas. There is no other abnormality within the abdomen.

5. What investigation would you require prior to obtaining the patient's consent for endoscopic retrograde cholangiopancreatography (ERCP)?

ERCP shows a stricture of the bile duct consistent with a carcinoma of the head of the pancreas.

6. What are the principles of management in this case and what operation might be considered?

3.1 INITIAL ASSESSMENT

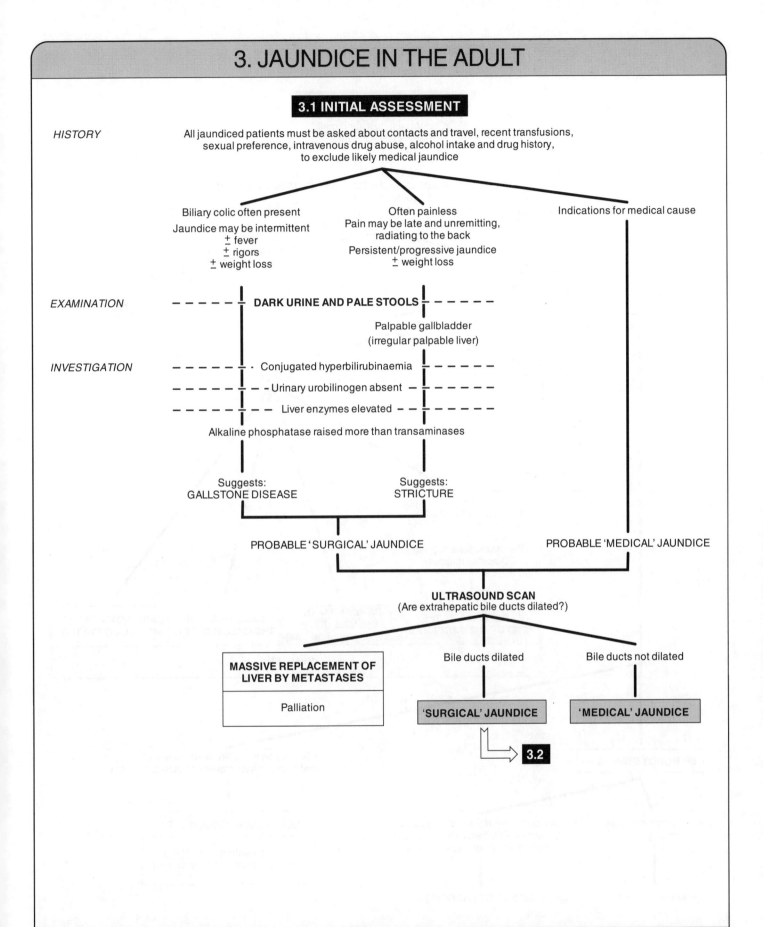

HISTORY

All jaundiced patients must be asked about contacts and travel, recent transfusions, sexual preference, intravenous drug abuse, alcohol intake and drug history, to exclude likely medical jaundice

Biliary colic often present

Jaundice may be intermittent
± fever
± rigors
± weight loss

Often painless
Pain may be late and unremitting, radiating to the back
Persistent/progressive jaundice
± weight loss

Indications for medical cause

EXAMINATION

DARK URINE AND PALE STOOLS

Palpable gallbladder
(irregular palpable liver)

INVESTIGATION

Conjugated hyperbilirubinaemia

Urinary urobilinogen absent

Liver enzymes elevated

Alkaline phosphatase raised more than transaminases

Suggests:
GALLSTONE DISEASE

Suggests:
STRICTURE

PROBABLE 'SURGICAL' JAUNDICE

PROBABLE 'MEDICAL' JAUNDICE

ULTRASOUND SCAN
(Are extrahepatic bile ducts dilated?)

MASSIVE REPLACEMENT OF LIVER BY METASTASES
Palliation

Bile ducts dilated

Bile ducts not dilated

'SURGICAL' JAUNDICE

'MEDICAL' JAUNDICE

3.2

3. JAUNDICE IN THE ADULT

3.2 SURGICAL JAUNDICE

Correct clotting if abnormal
Treat sepsis if present

ENDOSCOPIC RETROGRADE CHOLANGIOPANCREATOGRAPHY (ERCP)
± brushings/biopsy
Percutaneous transhepatic cholangiography (PTC) may be a useful adjunct to the difficult ERCP
It is still sometimes used alone where ERCP is not available

STRICTURE

GALLSTONES

3.3

Benign

Malignant

Secondary

Primary

SECONDARIES IN THE PORTA HEPATIS
Palliation

May be associated with:
– Thrombophlebitis migrans
– Acute pancreatitis
– Pancreatic steatorrhoea
– Diabetes mellitus

CARCINOMA OF THE HEAD OF THE PANCREAS	**CARCINOMA OF THE BILE DUCT (cholangiocarcinoma)**	**CARCINOMA OF THE GALLBLADDER**	**CARCINOMA OF THE AMPULLA OF VATER**
See p. 18			

BILE DUCT STENOSIS

Biliary tree looks like 'a tree in winter'
One-third of cases associated with ulcerative colitis

Previous instrumentation or surgery

Associated with acute cholecystitis
Oedema in enlarged gallbladder wall
compressing common bile duct

SCLEROSING CHOLANGITIS
Medical treatment is first line Liver transplant may be indicated

Stent or reoperate

MIRIZZI'S SYNDROME

3.3 GALLSTONES IN BILIARY TREE

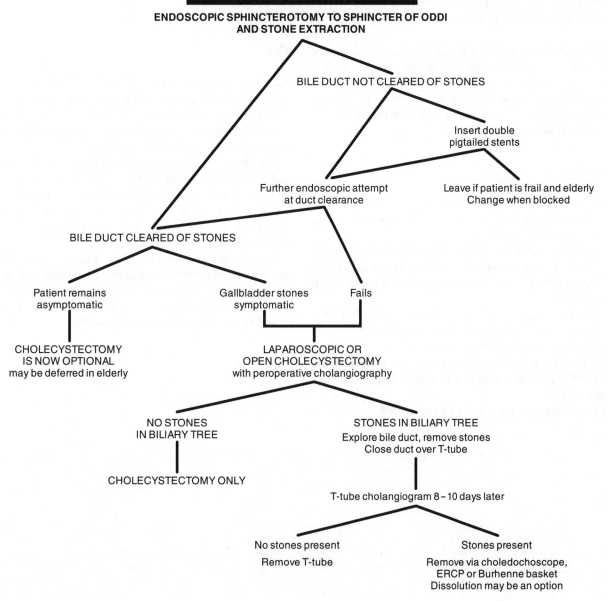

ENDOSCOPIC SPHINCTEROTOMY TO SPHINCTER OF ODDI AND STONE EXTRACTION

BILE DUCT NOT CLEARED OF STONES

Insert double pigtailed stents

Further endoscopic attempt at duct clearance

Leave if patient is frail and elderly
Change when blocked

BILE DUCT CLEARED OF STONES

Patient remains asymptomatic

Gallbladder stones symptomatic

Fails

CHOLECYSTECTOMY IS NOW OPTIONAL
may be deferred in elderly

LAPAROSCOPIC OR OPEN CHOLECYSTECTOMY
with peroperative cholangiography

NO STONES IN BILIARY TREE

STONES IN BILIARY TREE
Explore bile duct, remove stones
Close duct over T-tube

CHOLECYSTECTOMY ONLY

T-tube cholangiogram 8 – 10 days later

No stones present
Remove T-tube

Stones present
Remove via choledochoscope,
ERCP or Burhenne basket
Dissolution may be an option

PRINCIPLES OF THE TREATMENT OF MALIGNANT JAUNDICE

Surgery is the only curative modality – but the operative mortality is in general high and the long-term survival very poor (except in carcinoma of the ampulla). Ask yourself in each case whether the benefits justify the costs of attempted cure. Then decide whether to attempt cure or palliation.

Palliation

The usual aim of palliation is to relieve jaundice. The techniques are broadly similar for all causes of malignant obstructive jaundice.

Stenting at ERCP is relatively safe although in the long term the stents may become blocked and the bile infected (cholangitis). The stent may be changed when this occurs.

Palliative surgical biliary bypass has a much higher mortality (cholecystojejunostomy, choledochojejunostomy) but the incidence of recurrent jaundice and sepsis is lower. Late pyloric obstruction in carcinoma of the head of the pancreas may need surgical bypass (gastrojejunostomy).

Pain, where present, must be controlled.

Cure

Carcinoma of the head of the pancreas is the commonest of these malignancies. If the tumour is small and confined to the head with no metastases a very few may be cured by Whipple's operation – pancreatoduodenectomy – best done by a specialist surgeon.

Cholangiocarcinoma is slow-growing so that the results of palliation are good. A few localized tumours may be cured by resection, best done in a specialist unit.

Carcinoma of the gallbladder presents late and is generally only curable when so small that it is found coincidentally at cholecystectomy.

Carcinoma of the ampulla has a much better prognosis than all the above – if there is no evidence of spread on preoperative evaluation and the patient is fit then about 40% survive 5 years after pancreatoduodenectomy. Local resection is sometimes possible.

4. DYSPHAGIA

INTRODUCTION

Dysphagia or difficulty in swallowing is commonly caused by a narrowing of the lumen of the oesophagus (i.e. a structural cause) or oesophageal neuromuscular incoordination.

The structural causes may be:

a. a foreign body in the lumen of the oesophagus
b. oesophageal wall narrowing
c. external compression of the oesophagus

The following case history illustrates the work-up of a typical case of dysphagia.

Case history

An 83-year-old man presents complaining of an inability to swallow. This has been troubling him for 4 months and his intake is now restricted to fluids or mashed food. He has lost 12 kg in the last 3 months.

1. Does this history favour a benign or a malignant cause of dysphagia?

2. What investigation would be most likely to provide you with the diagnosis?

Upper gastrointestinal endoscopy reveals a malignant-looking stricture and a biopsy is taken.

3. What histologically differentiates carcinoma of the oesophagus from carcinoma of the stomach and cardia?

4. Why is this differentiation important?

The histology of this lesion is a squamous cell carcinoma.

An ultrasound of the liver reveals an irregularly enlarged liver with multiple spots of different echogenicity within its substance.

5. Is this tumour likely to be radiosensitive?

6. Would you attempt a curative procedure in this man?

7. How may his dysphagia be relieved?

4. DYSPHAGIA

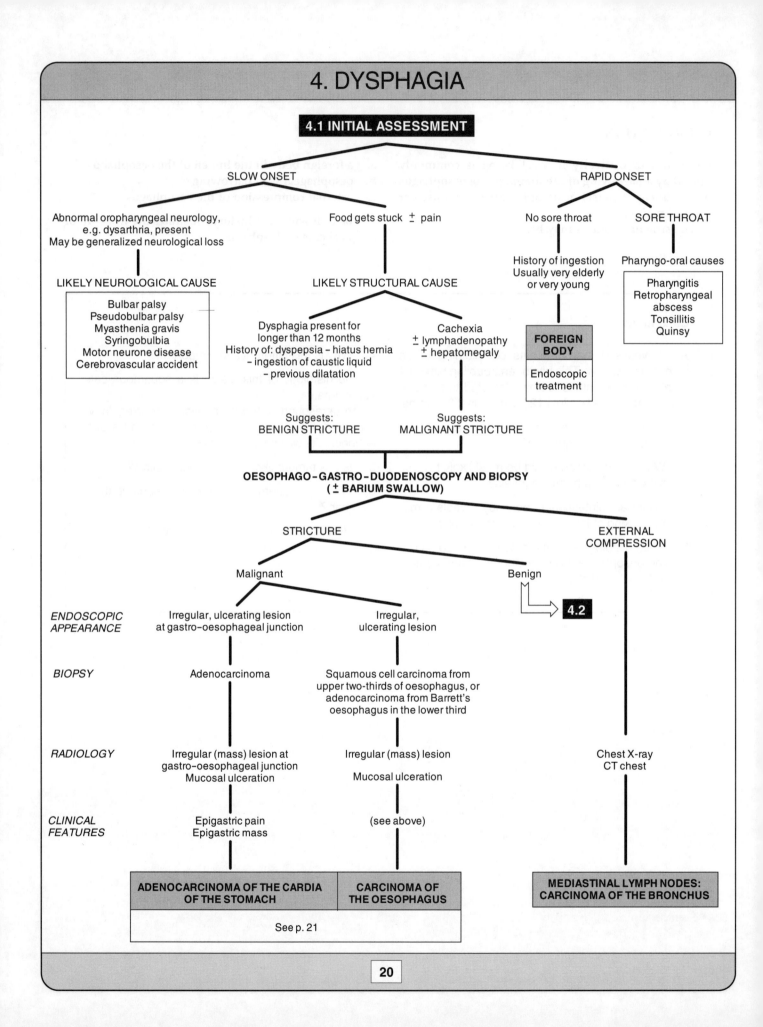

4.1 INITIAL ASSESSMENT

SLOW ONSET

RAPID ONSET

Abnormal oropharyngeal neurology,
e.g. dysarthria, present
May be generalized neurological loss

Food gets stuck ± pain

No sore throat

SORE THROAT

LIKELY NEUROLOGICAL CAUSE

Bulbar palsy
Pseudobulbar palsy
Myasthenia gravis
Syringobulbia
Motor neurone disease
Cerebrovascular accident

LIKELY STRUCTURAL CAUSE

Dysphagia present for
longer than 12 months
History of: dyspepsia – hiatus hernia
– ingestion of caustic liquid
– previous dilatation

Cachexia
± lymphadenopathy
± hepatomegaly

History of ingestion
Usually very elderly
or very young

Pharyngo-oral causes

Pharyngitis
Retropharyngeal
abscess
Tonsillitis
Quinsy

FOREIGN BODY

Endoscopic
treatment

Suggests:
BENIGN STRICTURE

Suggests:
MALIGNANT STRICTURE

OESOPHAGO–GASTRO–DUODENOSCOPY AND BIOPSY (± BARIUM SWALLOW)

STRICTURE

EXTERNAL COMPRESSION

Malignant

Benign → **4.2**

ENDOSCOPIC APPEARANCE

Irregular, ulcerating lesion
at gastro–oesophageal junction

Irregular,
ulcerating lesion

BIOPSY

Adenocarcinoma

Squamous cell carcinoma from
upper two-thirds of oesophagus, or
adenocarcinoma from Barrett's
oesophagus in the lower third

RADIOLOGY

Irregular (mass) lesion at
gastro–oesophageal junction
Mucosal ulceration

Irregular (mass) lesion

Mucosal ulceration

Chest X-ray
CT chest

CLINICAL FEATURES

Epigastric pain
Epigastric mass

(see above)

ADENOCARCINOMA OF THE CARDIA OF THE STOMACH

CARCINOMA OF THE OESOPHAGUS

MEDIASTINAL LYMPH NODES: CARCINOMA OF THE BRONCHUS

See p. 21

4. DYSPHAGIA

4.2 BENIGN STRICTURE

ENDOSCOPIC FINDINGS	Very dilated oesophagus proximal to a constricted lower oesophageal sphincter	Oesophageal ulceration or inflammation	Rarer differential diagnosis
			Plummer–Vinson or Patterson–Kelly–Brown syndrome Scleroderma Pharyngeal pouch Corkscrew oesophagus
BARIUM SWALLOW	Barium shows a 'mega-oesophagus' with tapering of the lower end 'widow's peak'		
CLINICAL FEATURES	Usually aged 20–40 years Symptoms may have been present for a long time May be retrosternal discomfort, fetid flatulence or aspiration pneumonitis	Reflux oesophagitis/heartburn Waterbrash	
TREATMENT	**ACHALASIA OF THE CARDIA** Dilatation of the sphincter using a Negus hydrostatic bag Surgery: Heller's cardiomyotomy	**PEPTIC STRICTURE ± OESOPHAGITIS ± HIATUS HERNIA** Dilate the stricture Prevent recurrence Conservative: – stop smoking, lose weight, avoid alcohol, elevate head of bed – antacids, H_2-blockers, proton-pump inhibitors Operations: – Nissen fundoplication – Angelchik prosthesis	

TREATMENT OF CARCINOMA OF THE STOMACH OR OESOPHAGUS CAUSING DYSPHAGIA

Regardless of treatment, the chances of surviving these disorders are very poor. 'Curative' operations are rarely possible – and when they are, they not only cause a high morbidity and mortality but rarely succeed in curing the patient. It is therefore important to decide for each patient whether the costs of curative procedures justify the benefits. The success of curative surgery depends on very careful patient selection.

Cure

Squamous cell carcinoma may be cured by surgery or radiotherapy. To date there is no clear difference in the reported survival of patients treated with either of these. Adenocarcinoma may only be cured by surgery. The surgical objectives are resection of tumour and its lymphatic drainage and replacement with stomach, jejunum or colon.

Palliation

Total dysphagia with an inability to swallow sputum is a very distressing symptom. Its relief is therefore the main aim of palliation. Stenting at gastroscopy is relatively safe although in the long term the stents may become blocked and the dysphagia returns. The stent may be changed when this occurs. Surgical bypass has a minor role in the palliation of dysphagia. Radiotherapy may be helpful although initially dysphagia may worsen. Remember, other aspects of good palliative care such as analgesia are very important.

5. HAEMATEMESIS AND MELAENA

Haematemesis is the symptom of vomiting blood, and commonly occurs as a result of upper gastrointestinal bleeding proximal to the pylorus. The blood may be altered dark red and of low volume, or fresh, red and enough to cause shock. It is a common presenting complaint to casualty departments and is managed by both physicians and surgeons.

Melaena is the passage of dark (often black), offensive, altered bloody faeces per rectum. It is caused by upper gastrointestinal bleeding. It is often difficult to differentiate clinically between melaena and altered blood in the stool from a colorectal bleed. Similarly, torrential upper GI bleeding, presenting as the passage of red blood per rectum, may be mistaken as rectal in origin. The lines of investigation for each of these conditions are considered in this chapter and Chapter 6.

5. HAEMATEMESIS AND MELAENA

5.1 INITIAL ASSESSMENT

Low volume loss
Patient haemodynamically stable
ROUTINE ASSESSMENT

Tachycardia, low volume pulse
Hypotension, low urine output
Drowsiness, sweating, pallor

HYPOTENSIVE SHOCK
1. IMMEDIATE RESUSCITATION
   Oxygen by mask, i.v. access, urinary catheter and nasogastric tube
2. I.V. VOLUME REPLACEMENT
   with colloid/crystalloid (not dextrose) titrated against blood pressure, CVP and urine output
3. FBC, U&E, G&S and cross-match

SUCCESSFUL
RESUSCITATION

FAILURE OF
RESUSCITATION

Stable patient

Indicates uncontrolled
haemorrhage

LAPAROTOMY

CLINICAL FEATURES

Ask about aetiological factors of hepatic cirrhosis,
e.g. alcohol and/or drug abuse,
hepatitis B infections

Clinical features of chronic liver disease:
'liver palms'/'flap', jaundice, fetor, anaemia,
spider naevi, gynaecomastia, ascites,
'caput medusae', testicular atrophy

Encephalopathy

Portal hypertension

Suggests:
VARICEAL BLEEDING

Epigastric pain
Anorexia
Weight loss
Anaemia
Epigastric mass
Virchow node

History of smoking, alcohol abuse

Pernicious anaemia

Suggests:
CARCINOMA

Retrosternal pain/discomfort,
worse on bending, lying down
Suggests: Oesophageal site

Postprandial epigastric pain/discomfort
dissuades from eating
Suggests: Gastric site

Preprandial upper abdominal pain,
relieved by milk/antacids
Suggests: Duodenal site

Relieved by antacids/H_2-blockers
History of smoking, NSAID or alcohol abuse

Suggests:
BENIGN ULCERATION

'Nil by mouth' on i.v. fluid replacement until

OESOPHAGO-GASTRO-DUODENOSCOPY (OGD) ON NEXT AVAILABLE ENDOSCOPY LIST

Aim to see the whole of the upper gastrointestinal tract if possible;
oesophageal varices do not preclude bleeding from a peptic ulcer

BLOOD TRANSFUSION MAY BE REQUIRED

OESOPHAGEAL LESION   **GASTRIC LESION**   **DUODENAL LESION**

5.2   5.3   5.4

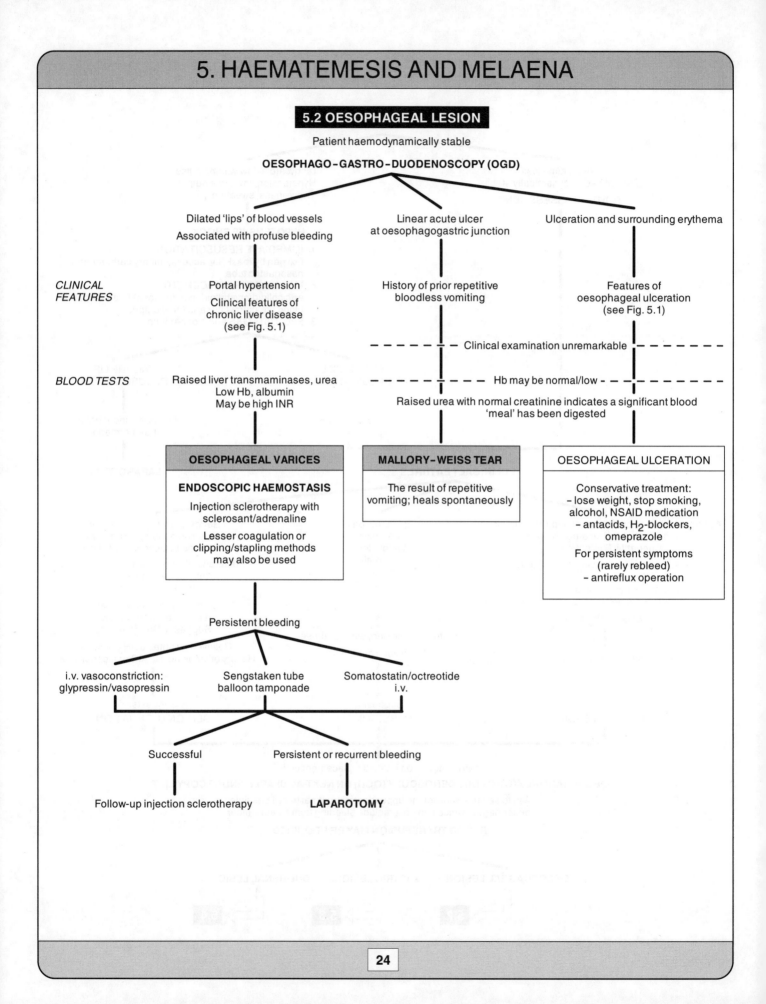

5.2 OESOPHAGEAL LESION

Patient haemodynamically stable

OESOPHAGO – GASTRO – DUODENOSCOPY (OGD)

| Dilated 'lips' of blood vessels | Linear acute ulcer | Ulceration and surrounding erythema |
| Associated with profuse bleeding | at oesophagogastric junction | |

CLINICAL FEATURES

Portal hypertension

Clinical features of chronic liver disease (see Fig. 5.1)

History of prior repetitive bloodless vomiting

Features of oesophageal ulceration (see Fig. 5.1)

Clinical examination unremarkable

BLOOD TESTS

Raised liver transmaminases, urea Low Hb, albumin May be high INR

Hb may be normal/low

Raised urea with normal creatinine indicates a significant blood 'meal' has been digested

OESOPHAGEAL VARICES

ENDOSCOPIC HAEMOSTASIS

Injection sclerotherapy with sclerosant/adrenaline

Lesser coagulation or clipping/stapling methods may also be used

MALLORY – WEISS TEAR

The result of repetitive vomiting; heals spontaneously

OESOPHAGEAL ULCERATION

Conservative treatment:
– lose weight, stop smoking, alcohol, NSAID medication
– antacids, H_2-blockers, omeprazole

For persistent symptoms (rarely rebleed)
– antireflux operation

Persistent bleeding

| i.v. vasoconstriction: glypressin/vasopressin | Sengstaken tube balloon tamponade | Somatostatin/octreotide i.v. |

Successful

Persistent or recurrent bleeding

Follow-up injection sclerotherapy

LAPAROTOMY

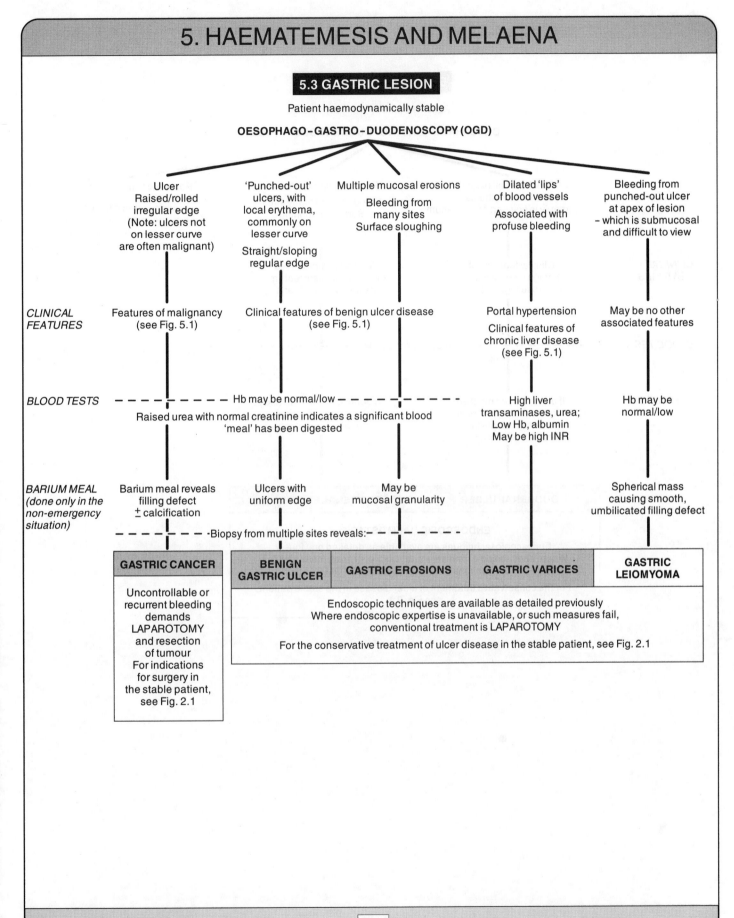

5.3 GASTRIC LESION

Patient haemodynamically stable

OESOPHAGO - GASTRO - DUODENOSCOPY (OGD)

	Ulcer Raised/rolled irregular edge (Note: ulcers not on lesser curve are often malignant)	'Punched-out' ulcers, with local erythema, commonly on lesser curve Straight/sloping regular edge	Multiple mucosal erosions Bleeding from many sites Surface sloughing	Dilated 'lips' of blood vessels Associated with profuse bleeding	Bleeding from punched-out ulcer at apex of lesion – which is submucosal and difficult to view
CLINICAL FEATURES	Features of malignancy (see Fig. 5.1)	Clinical features of benign ulcer disease (see Fig. 5.1)		Portal hypertension Clinical features of chronic liver disease (see Fig. 5.1)	May be no other associated features
BLOOD TESTS	Hb may be normal/low — Raised urea with normal creatinine indicates a significant blood 'meal' has been digested			High liver transaminases, urea; Low Hb, albumin May be high INR	Hb may be normal/low
BARIUM MEAL (done only in the non-emergency situation)	Barium meal reveals filling defect ± calcification	Ulcers with uniform edge	May be mucosal granularity		Spherical mass causing smooth, umbilicated filling defect
	Biopsy from multiple sites reveals:				

GASTRIC CANCER	**BENIGN GASTRIC ULCER**	**GASTRIC EROSIONS**	**GASTRIC VARICES**	**GASTRIC LEIOMYOMA**
Uncontrollable or recurrent bleeding demands LAPAROTOMY and resection of tumour For indications for surgery in the stable patient, see Fig. 2.1	Endoscopic techniques are available as detailed previously Where endoscopic expertise is unavailable, or such measures fail, conventional treatment is LAPAROTOMY For the conservative treatment of ulcer disease in the stable patient, see Fig. 2.1			

5.4 DUODENAL LESION

Patient haemodynamically stable

OESOPHAGO – GASTRO – DUODENOSCOPY (OGD)

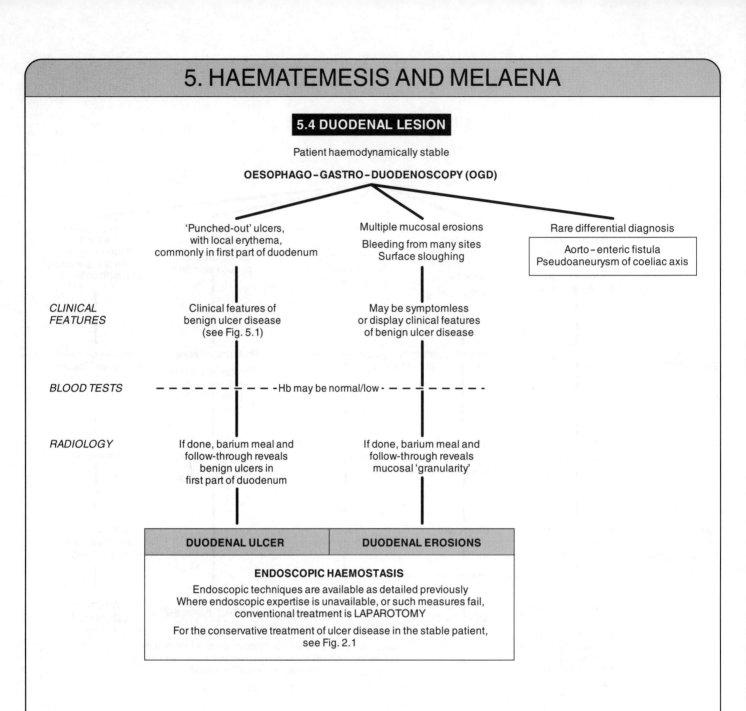

'Punched-out' ulcers,
with local erythema,
commonly in first part of duodenum

Multiple mucosal erosions
Bleeding from many sites
Surface sloughing

Rare differential diagnosis

Aorto – enteric fistula
Pseudoaneurysm of coeliac axis

CLINICAL FEATURES

Clinical features of
benign ulcer disease
(see Fig. 5.1)

May be symptomless
or display clinical features
of benign ulcer disease

BLOOD TESTS — — — — — — — — Hb may be normal/low — — — — — — —

RADIOLOGY

If done, barium meal and
follow-through reveals
benign ulcers in
first part of duodenum

If done, barium meal and
follow-through reveals
mucosal 'granularity'

DUODENAL ULCER	DUODENAL EROSIONS

ENDOSCOPIC HAEMOSTASIS

Endoscopic techniques are available as detailed previously
Where endoscopic expertise is unavailable, or such measures fail,
conventional treatment is LAPAROTOMY

For the conservative treatment of ulcer disease in the stable patient,
see Fig. 2.1

6. BLEEDING PER RECTUM

INTRODUCTION

The source of rectal bleeding may be anywhere along the length of the gastrointestinal tract, and thus a careful clinical evaluation is important, governing the choice of appropriate investigations. Rectal bleeding should not be confused with melaena, for which see Chapter 5. Other chapters of relevance are Chapters 7 and 8.

Case history

A 30-year-old woman is referred to surgical out-patients with a 1-week history of bloody and offensive diarrhoea. She has lost her appetite, feels generally weak and unwell and complains of crampy, episodic, left-sided abdominal pain. Her bowels open up to 15 times a day, with a sensation of urgency. On examination she is thin, fluid-depleted and unwell. She is clinically anaemic and has a soft, non-tender abdomen and normal rectal examination. Her past medical history contains an episode of deep venous thrombosis, for which she is currently being given warfarin.

1. What are the clinical diagnoses suggested and what should be the first examination?

   Sigmoidoscopy reveals an inflamed, thin and friable mucosa with contact bleeding. No mass lesion is seen.

2. Under the circumstances, what would deter you from biopsy of the mucosa?

   In view of the fragile state of the mucosa the surgeon decides against biopsy because of the risk of perforation during the planned barium enema. Furthermore, the patient is anticoagulated, providing a relative contraindication to outpatient biopsy.

3. What further investigations would confirm the diagnosis?

   The patient is admitted from the clinic. Barium enema reveals mucosal ulceration and granularity. The bowel is dilated and displays pseudopolyps. The abnormality is continuous from the rectum proximally and blood tests confirm an anaemia, mild leukocytosis, raised ESR and low albumin.

4. What are the most likely diagnoses and how would you differentiate between them?

   The differential diagnosis of ulcerative colitis or Crohn's disease is made, and the surgeon plans a colonoscopy and biopsy. The biopsy reveals a non-granulomatous mucosal dystrophy with chronic inflammation.

5. What is the diagnosis, and what factors would govern the surgeon's decision to operate in the stable patient?

6. BLEEDING PER RECTUM

6.1 INITIAL ASSESSMENT

Correct clotting if abnormal

Bright red or altered blood mixed with stool	Bright red bleeding; fresh blood drips in pan, or covering stool, paper	Dark black stool; may be offensive, tarry diarrhoea – melaena
May be lower abdominal colic (hindgut) or rectal pain/tenesmus	± Anal pain or discomfort	History of haematemesis
± Urgent and frequent defaecation ± Change in bowel habit ± Mucus/pus per rectum	± Anal pruritus	May be central abdominal pain (midgut)
RECTAL OR COLONIC HAEMORRHAGE ↳ **6.3**	**ANAL OR LOW RECTAL HAEMORRHAGE**	**UPPER GASTROINTESTINAL TRACT HAEMORRHAGE** ↳ **Ch. 5**

Painful   Painless ↳ **6.2**

Pain at anal margin, much worse on and after defaecation History of constipation	Pain unrelated to defaecation	Pain/rectal cramp Urgent and frequent defaecation
ON EXAMINATION	ON EXAMINATION	ON EXAMINATION
Exquisitely tender mucocutaneous tear in posterior midline anus (may be anterior in female patient)	Ulcerated, indurated anal mass Palpable on rectal examination	Rectal examination is normal
	Biopsy: squamous cell carcinoma	**SIGMOIDOSCOPY** Inflamed mucosa, with surface bleeding
		PROCTITIS

FISSURE-IN-ANO

Pain relief and stool softeners
Anal stretch under
general anaesthesia

ANAL CARCINOMA

Radiotherapy, chemotherapy

Operation if failure of above

BARIUM ENEMA

defines the extent and distribution
and identifies proximal lesions

Biopsy and stool culture

For multiple fissures in odd sites
Consider cause:

Crohn's disease
Carcinoma
Tuberculosis

INFECTIVE PROCTITIS

Treat infection and
maintain fluid balance

CROHN'S COLITIS	ULCERATIVE COLITIS
See p. 41	

6. BLEEDING PER RECTUM

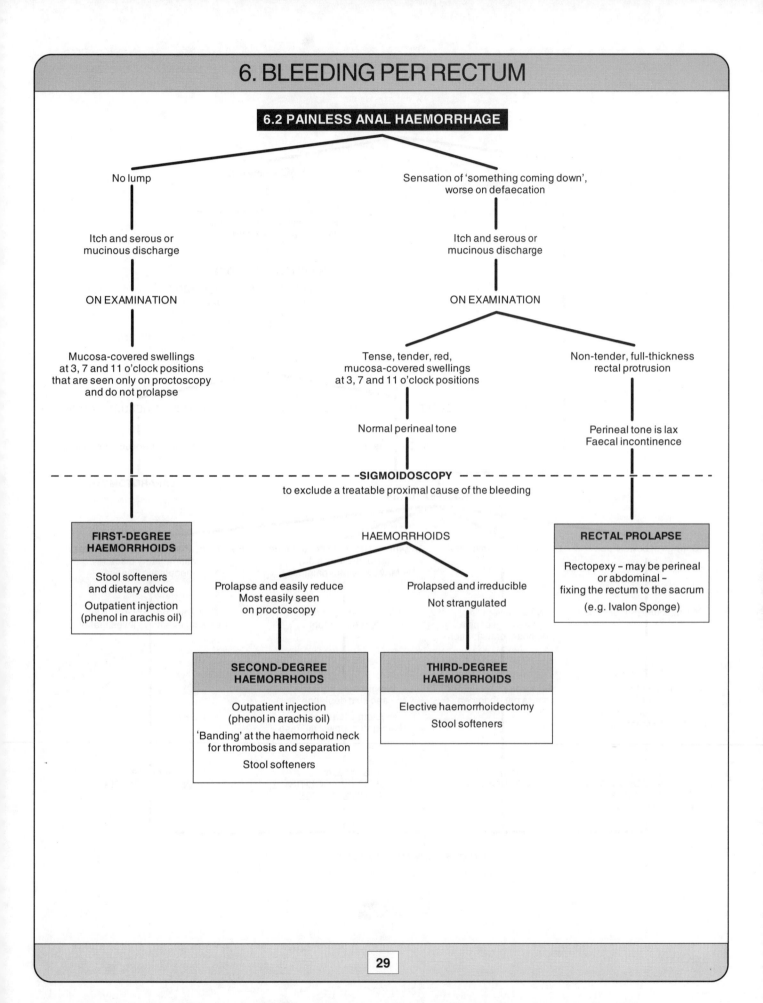

6.2 PAINLESS ANAL HAEMORRHAGE

No lump

Sensation of 'something coming down', worse on defaecation

Itch and serous or mucinous discharge

Itch and serous or mucinous discharge

ON EXAMINATION

ON EXAMINATION

Mucosa-covered swellings at 3, 7 and 11 o'clock positions that are seen only on proctoscopy and do not prolapse

Tense, tender, red, mucosa-covered swellings at 3, 7 and 11 o'clock positions

Non-tender, full-thickness rectal protrusion

Normal perineal tone

Perineal tone is lax
Faecal incontinence

– – – SIGMOIDOSCOPY – – –
to exclude a treatable proximal cause of the bleeding

FIRST-DEGREE HAEMORRHOIDS

Stool softeners and dietary advice

Outpatient injection (phenol in arachis oil)

HAEMORRHOIDS

RECTAL PROLAPSE

Rectopexy – may be perineal or abdominal – fixing the rectum to the sacrum

(e.g. Ivalon Sponge)

Prolapse and easily reduce
Most easily seen on proctoscopy

Prolapsed and irreducible
Not strangulated

SECOND-DEGREE HAEMORRHOIDS

Outpatient injection (phenol in arachis oil)

'Banding' at the haemorrhoid neck for thrombosis and separation

Stool softeners

THIRD-DEGREE HAEMORRHOIDS

Elective haemorrhoidectomy

Stool softeners

6. BLEEDING PER RECTUM

6.3 COLONIC HAEMORRHAGE (1)

Low volume loss
Patient haemodynamically stable

ROUTINE ASSESSMENT

Large volume loss

Tachycardia, low volume pulse
Hypotension, low urine output
Drowsiness, sweating, pallor

HYPOTENSIVE SHOCK

1. IMMEDIATE RESUSCITATION
   Oxygen by mask, i.v. access, urinary catheter and
   nasogastric tube
2. I.V. VOLUME REPLACEMENT
   with colloid/crystalloid (not dextrose) titrated against
   blood pressure, CVP and urine output
3. FBC, U&E, G&S and cross-match

SUCCESSFUL RESUSCITATION

Stable patient

FAILURE OF RESUSCITATION

Indicates uncontrolled haemorrhage

LAPAROTOMY

CLINICAL FEATURES

Change of bowel habit	Left-sided abdominal pain	Urgent and frequent defaecation: up to 20 times a day. May be painful/painless	Persistent anaemia, with no features of: – inflammatory disease – neoplastic disease
Mucus/slime per rectum	Nausea, vomiting, 'flatulent dyspepsia' Diarrhoea, constipation	Mucus/slime per rectum ± Bloody stool	Often diagnosis of exclusion following extensive investigation
May be mass per abdomen or Palpable rectal mass May be tenesmus	May be palpable tender mass per abdomen	Weight loss, anorexia and fluid depletion Systemic features of inflammatory bowel disease	
Suggests: RECTAL/COLONIC ADENOCARCINOMA OR LARGE ADENOMA	Suggests: DIVERTICULITIS	Suggests: ULCERATIVE COLITIS CROHN'S COLITIS	Suggests: ANGIODYSPLASIA

SIGMOIDOSCOPY AND BIOPSY

(Flexible sigmoidoscopy reaches splenic flexure)

→ **5.3**

6.4 COLONIC HAEMORRHAGE (2)

SIGMOIDOSCOPY AND BIOPSY
(Flexible sigmoidoscopy reaches splenic flexure)

Normal

Polypoid, stenosing or
ulcerated mass lesion
Polyps may be multiple

Inflammation and
mucosal bleeding

May be constipated bowel
loaded with faeces

Defer biopsy if barium enema to be done within 2 weeks
because of risk of perforation

COLITIS

**DOUBLE-CONTRAST BARIUM ENEMA AND/OR
COLONOSCOPY AND BIOPSY**

RADIOLOGY
(in the stable
patient)

Irregular filling
defects,
e.g. 'apple-core'
lesion
Stricture

Any number
of smooth
filling defects

Diverticula
± strictures

Normal

Colitis

6.5

ENDOSCOPY

Polypoid, stenosing or ulcerated mass lesion
Polyps may be multiple
May be mucus ++

Chronic inflammation
and diverticula

Vascular
malformation
amid normal mucosa

Normal

6.6

BIOPSY

Adenocarcinoma

Adenoma

Benign inflammation

RECTAL/COLONIC ADENOCARCINOMA	BENIGN ADENOMA	DIVERTICULAR DISEASE	ANGIODYSPLASIA
See p. 41	Premalignant Multiple in time and space Colonoscopic snare and removal, with regular follow-up	Resuscitate When stable, conservative treatment with stool softeners and dietary advice	Embolization under radiological control Diathermy coagulation at colonoscopy May require resection of affected bowel

6.5 COLONIC HAEMORRHAGE (3) – COLITIS

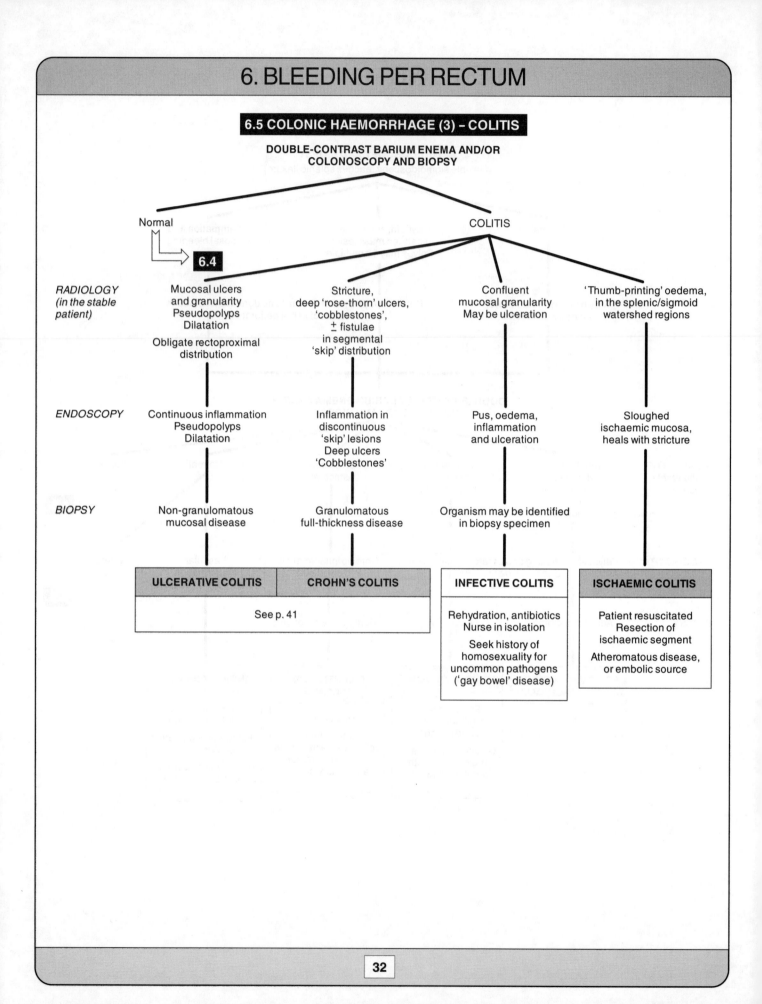

DOUBLE-CONTRAST BARIUM ENEMA AND/OR COLONOSCOPY AND BIOPSY

Normal → **6.4**

COLITIS

RADIOLOGY (in the stable patient)	Mucosal ulcers and granularity Pseudopolyps Dilatation Obligate rectoproximal distribution	Stricture, deep 'rose-thorn' ulcers, 'cobblestones', ± fistulae in segmental 'skip' distribution	Confluent mucosal granularity May be ulceration	'Thumb-printing' oedema, in the splenic/sigmoid watershed regions
ENDOSCOPY	Continuous inflammation Pseudopolyps Dilatation	Inflammation in discontinuous 'skip' lesions Deep ulcers 'Cobblestones'	Pus, oedema, inflammation and ulceration	Sloughed ischaemic mucosa, heals with stricture
BIOPSY	Non-granulomatous mucosal disease	Granulomatous full-thickness disease	Organism may be identified in biopsy specimen	

ULCERATIVE COLITIS	CROHN'S COLITIS	INFECTIVE COLITIS	ISCHAEMIC COLITIS
See p. 41		Rehydration, antibiotics Nurse in isolation Seek history of homosexuality for uncommon pathogens ('gay bowel' disease)	Patient resuscitated Resection of ischaemic segment Atheromatous disease, or embolic source

6.6 COLONIC HAEMORRHAGE (4)

Sigmoidoscopy, barium enema and colonoscopy
all fail to reveal bleeding point, and symptoms persist

No suspicion of upper gastrointestinal
source of bleeding
or
upper gastrointestinal investigations
normal

Consider:

ANGIOGRAPHY
Superior and inferior
mesenteric arteries
and coeliac axis

**TECHNETIUM-LABELLED
RED CELL SCANNING**

Both these investigations depend upon active bleeding
at the time of investigation
A negative result does not disprove the diagnosis

Abnormal

Identifies bleeding site

Labelled red blood cell
'leak' into lumen
is identified

Suspicion of upper gastrointestinal
source of bleeding

High blood urea on serum sampling
suggests high volume 'blood meal'

UPPER GASTROINTESTINAL ENDOSCOPY

→ **5.1**

If both these investigations prove unfruitful
in the face of continued bleeding, LAPAROTOMY
with on-table whole-bowel ENTEROSCOPY
may be considered

ARTERIOVENOUS MALFORMATION	**ANGIODYSPLASIA**
Embolization under radiological control Diathermy coagulation at colonoscopy May require resection of affected bowel	

MECKEL'S DIVERTICULUM
Resection if symptoms persist

7. CHANGE OF BOWEL HABIT

This is an important symptom because many of these patients will have a colorectal cancer. A change in bowel habit is usually of insidious onset and may be either increasing constipation, increasing diarrhoea or alternate periods of diarrhoea and constipation. Acute diarrhoea and acute constipation are not considered in this chapter.

This chapter should be read in conjunction with Chapters 6 and 8.

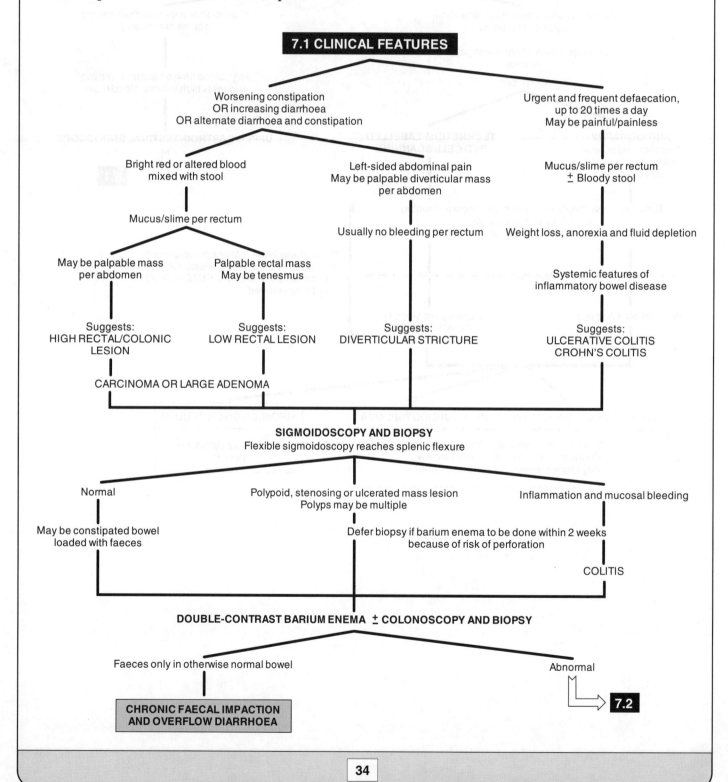

7.1 CLINICAL FEATURES

Worsening constipation
OR increasing diarrhoea
OR alternate diarrhoea and constipation

Urgent and frequent defaecation, up to 20 times a day
May be painful/painless

Bright red or altered blood mixed with stool

Left-sided abdominal pain
May be palpable diverticular mass per abdomen

Mucus/slime per rectum
± Bloody stool

Mucus/slime per rectum

Usually no bleeding per rectum

Weight loss, anorexia and fluid depletion

May be palpable mass per abdomen

Palpable rectal mass
May be tenesmus

Systemic features of inflammatory bowel disease

Suggests:
HIGH RECTAL/COLONIC LESION

Suggests:
LOW RECTAL LESION

Suggests:
DIVERTICULAR STRICTURE

Suggests:
ULCERATIVE COLITIS
CROHN'S COLITIS

CARCINOMA OR LARGE ADENOMA

SIGMOIDOSCOPY AND BIOPSY
Flexible sigmoidoscopy reaches splenic flexure

Normal

Polypoid, stenosing or ulcerated mass lesion
Polyps may be multiple

Inflammation and mucosal bleeding

May be constipated bowel loaded with faeces

Defer biopsy if barium enema to be done within 2 weeks because of risk of perforation

COLITIS

DOUBLE-CONTRAST BARIUM ENEMA ± COLONOSCOPY AND BIOPSY

Faeces only in otherwise normal bowel

Abnormal

CHRONIC FAECAL IMPACTION AND OVERFLOW DIARRHOEA

7.2

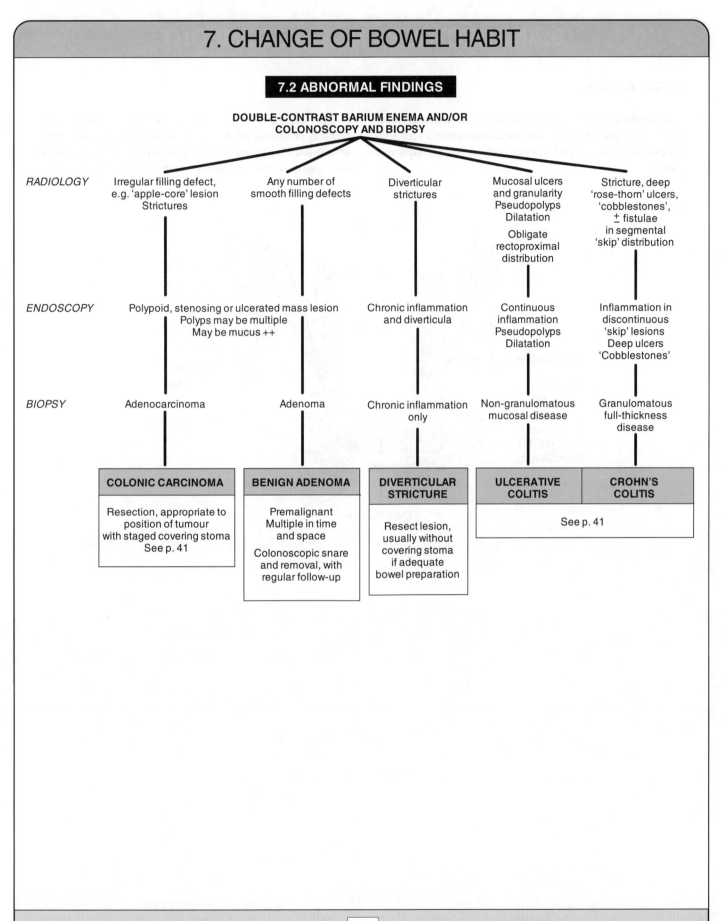

7.2 ABNORMAL FINDINGS

**DOUBLE-CONTRAST BARIUM ENEMA AND/OR
COLONOSCOPY AND BIOPSY**

RADIOLOGY

Irregular filling defect,
e.g. 'apple-core' lesion
Strictures

Any number of
smooth filling defects

Diverticular
strictures

Mucosal ulcers
and granularity
Pseudopolyps
Dilatation

Obligate
rectoproximal
distribution

Stricture, deep
'rose-thorn' ulcers,
'cobblestones',
± fistulae
in segmental
'skip' distribution

ENDOSCOPY

Polypoid, stenosing or ulcerated mass lesion
Polyps may be multiple
May be mucus ++

Chronic inflammation
and diverticula

Continuous
inflammation
Pseudopolyps
Dilatation

Inflammation in
discontinuous
'skip' lesions
Deep ulcers
'Cobblestones'

BIOPSY

Adenocarcinoma

Adenoma

Chronic inflammation
only

Non-granulomatous
mucosal disease

Granulomatous
full-thickness
disease

COLONIC CARCINOMA	BENIGN ADENOMA	DIVERTICULAR STRICTURE	ULCERATIVE COLITIS	CROHN'S COLITIS
Resection, appropriate to position of tumour with staged covering stoma See p. 41	Premalignant Multiple in time and space Colonoscopic snare and removal, with regular follow-up	Resect lesion, usually without covering stoma if adequate bowel preparation	See p. 41	

See p. 41

INTRODUCTION

A wide range of infective, inflammatory and neoplastic conditions present with anorectal symptoms and this chapter should be read in conjunction with Chapters 6 and 7.

The diagram below illustrates the important anatomical relations of the anal canal. Operations in this area must aim to preserve continence through minimal disruption of the sphincter mechanisms.

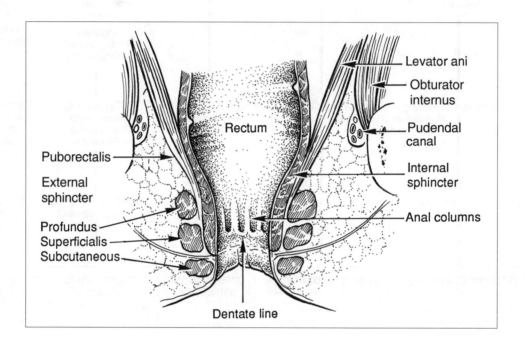

8. ANORECTAL PAIN OR DISCOMFORT

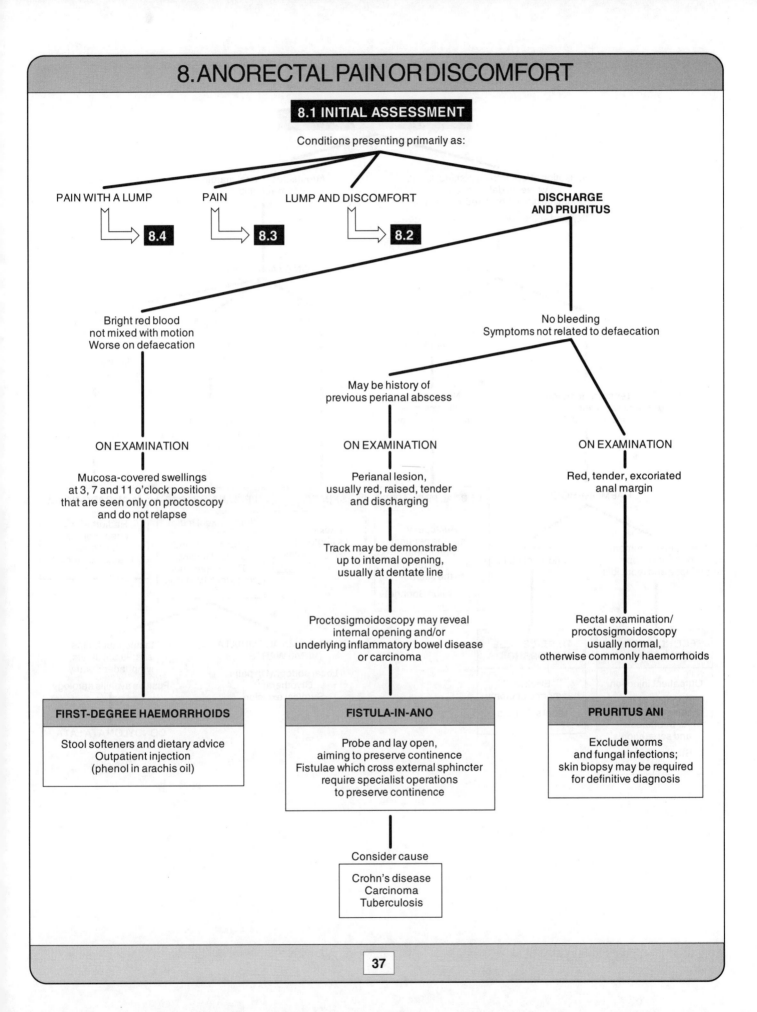

8.1 INITIAL ASSESSMENT

Conditions presenting primarily as:

PAIN WITH A LUMP → 8.4

PAIN → 8.3

LUMP AND DISCOMFORT → 8.2

DISCHARGE AND PRURITUS

Bright red blood
not mixed with motion
Worse on defaecation

No bleeding
Symptoms not related to defaecation

May be history of
previous perianal abscess

ON EXAMINATION

Mucosa-covered swellings
at 3, 7 and 11 o'clock positions
that are seen only on proctoscopy
and do not relapse

ON EXAMINATION

Perianal lesion,
usually red, raised, tender
and discharging

Track may be demonstrable
up to internal opening,
usually at dentate line

Proctosigmoidoscopy may reveal
internal opening and/or
underlying inflammatory bowel disease
or carcinoma

ON EXAMINATION

Red, tender, excoriated
anal margin

Rectal examination/
proctosigmoidoscopy
usually normal,
otherwise commonly haemorrhoids

FIRST-DEGREE HAEMORRHOIDS

Stool softeners and dietary advice
Outpatient injection
(phenol in arachis oil)

FISTULA-IN-ANO

Probe and lay open,
aiming to preserve continence
Fistulae which cross external sphincter
require specialist operations
to preserve continence

Consider cause

Crohn's disease
Carcinoma
Tuberculosis

PRURITUS ANI

Exclude worms
and fungal infections;
skin biopsy may be required
for definitive diagnosis

8.2 LUMP AND DISCOMFORT

Sensation of 'something coming down',
worse on defaecation
Bright red blood not mixed with motion

Itch and serous or mucinous discharge

ON EXAMINATION

Normal perineal tone

Perineal tone is lax
Faecal incontinence
in elderly woman

Tense, tender, red,
mucosa-covered swellings
at 3, 7 and 11 o'clock positions

Non-tender,
full-thickness
rectal protrusion

HAEMORRHOIDS

Seen most commonly
on proctoscopy;
prolapse and reducible

Prolapsed
and irreducible

RECTAL PROLAPSE

Rectopexy
– may be perineal
or abdominal –
fixing the rectum
to the sacrum

(e.g. Ivalon Sponge)

SECOND-DEGREE HAEMORRHOIDS

Outpatient injection

'Banding' at the
haemorrhoid neck
for thrombosis
and separation

Stool softeners

THIRD-DEGREE HAEMORRHOIDS

Elective
haemorrhoidectomy

Stool softeners

At/outside the anal margin
Non-reducible

ON EXAMINATION

Tag of skin

**Multiple,
pedunculated
papillomata
around anus**

**Hard, craggy mass,
continuous with
anal margin**

May be ulcerated,
bleeding and infected

May spread to
vagina/scrotum/penis
and into anal canal

Biopsy

Squamous cell
carcinoma

SKIN TAG

Excision
if symptoms
causing distress

PERIANAL WARTS
(usually
homosexual male)

Counselling and
contact tracing
STD screen and
consider HIV status

ANAL CARCINOMA

Radiotherapy,
chemotherapy
Operation
if failure of above

CONDYLOMA ACUMINATA
(VIRAL WARTS)

Local podophyllin paint
Cryotherapy
Surgical excision

Maculopapular rash,
snail-track ulcers,
lymphadenopathy

Positive syphilis serology

CONDYLOMATA LATA
(SYPHILIS)

Penicillin

8. ANORECTAL PAIN OR DISCOMFORT

8.3 PAIN

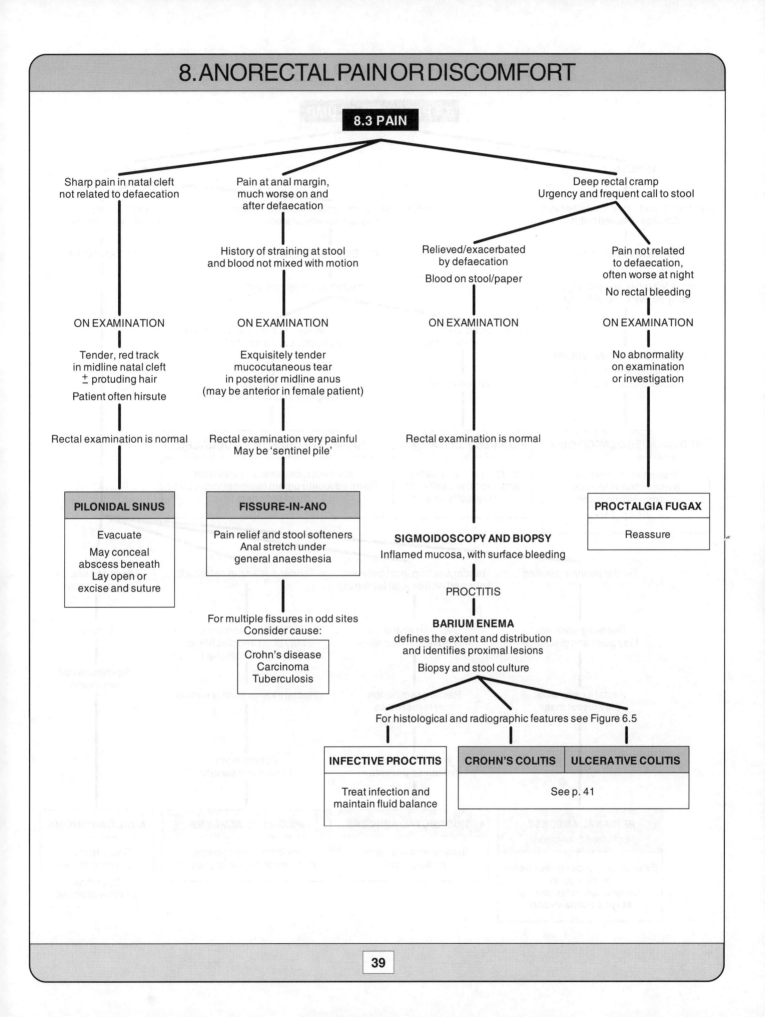

Sharp pain in natal cleft not related to defaecation

ON EXAMINATION

Tender, red track in midline natal cleft ± protuding hair

Patient often hirsute

Rectal examination is normal

PILONIDAL SINUS

Evacuate

May conceal abscess beneath Lay open or excise and suture

Pain at anal margin, much worse on and after defaecation

History of straining at stool and blood not mixed with motion

ON EXAMINATION

Exquisitely tender mucocutaneous tear in posterior midline anus (may be anterior in female patient)

Rectal examination very painful May be 'sentinel pile'

FISSURE-IN-ANO

Pain relief and stool softeners Anal stretch under general anaesthesia

For multiple fissures in odd sites Consider cause:

Crohn's disease
Carcinoma
Tuberculosis

Deep rectal cramp Urgency and frequent call to stool

Relieved/exacerbated by defaecation

Blood on stool/paper

ON EXAMINATION

Rectal examination is normal

SIGMOIDOSCOPY AND BIOPSY

Inflamed mucosa, with surface bleeding

PROCTITIS

BARIUM ENEMA

defines the extent and distribution and identifies proximal lesions

Biopsy and stool culture

For histological and radiographic features see Figure 6.5

INFECTIVE PROCTITIS

Treat infection and maintain fluid balance

CROHN'S COLITIS | ULCERATIVE COLITIS

See p. 41

Pain not related to defaecation, often worse at night

No rectal bleeding

ON EXAMINATION

No abnormality on examination or investigation

PROCTALGIA FUGAX

Reassure

8.4 PAIN WITH A LUMP

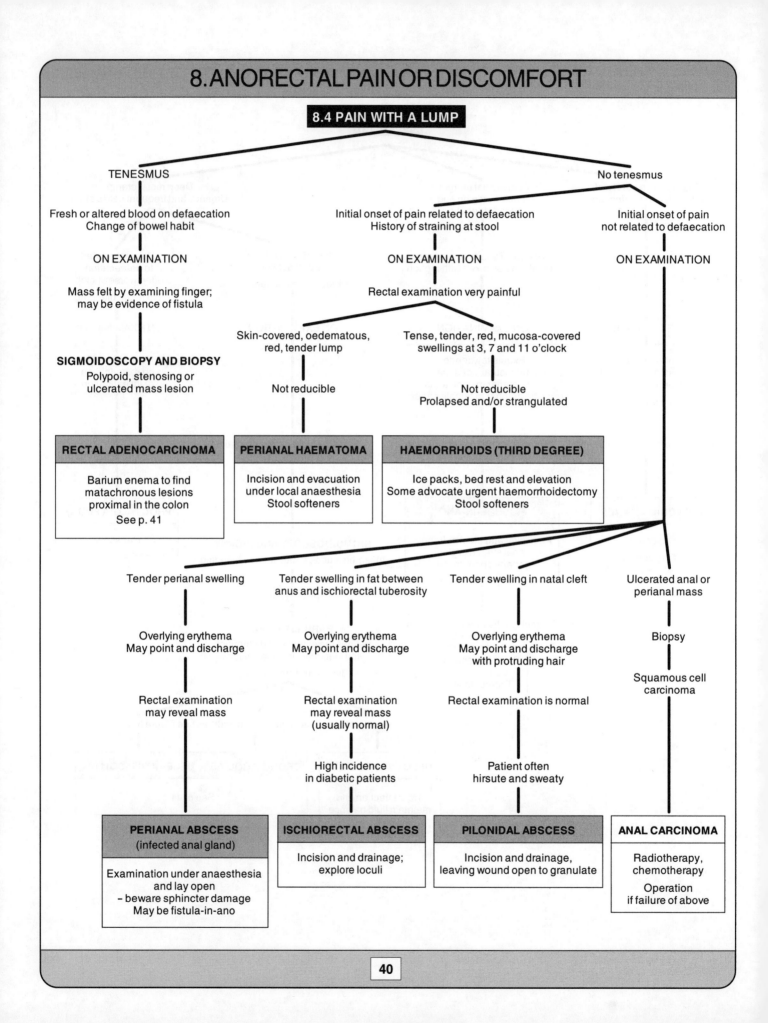

TENESMUS

Fresh or altered blood on defaecation
Change of bowel habit

ON EXAMINATION

Mass felt by examining finger;
may be evidence of fistula

SIGMOIDOSCOPY AND BIOPSY
Polypoid, stenosing or
ulcerated mass lesion

RECTAL ADENOCARCINOMA
Barium enema to find
matachronous lesions
proximal in the colon
See p. 41

No tenesmus

Initial onset of pain related to defaecation
History of straining at stool

ON EXAMINATION

Rectal examination very painful

Skin-covered, oedematous,
red, tender lump

Not reducible

PERIANAL HAEMATOMA
Incision and evacuation
under local anaesthesia
Stool softeners

Tense, tender, red, mucosa-covered
swellings at 3, 7 and 11 o'clock

Not reducible
Prolapsed and/or strangulated

HAEMORRHOIDS (THIRD DEGREE)
Ice packs, bed rest and elevation
Some advocate urgent haemorrhoidectomy
Stool softeners

Initial onset of pain
not related to defaecation

ON EXAMINATION

Tender perianal swelling

Overlying erythema
May point and discharge

Rectal examination
may reveal mass

PERIANAL ABSCESS
(infected anal gland)
Examination under anaesthesia
and lay open
– beware sphincter damage
May be fistula-in-ano

Tender swelling in fat between
anus and ischiorectal tuberosity

Overlying erythema
May point and discharge

Rectal examination
may reveal mass
(usually normal)

High incidence
in diabetic patients

ISCHIORECTAL ABSCESS
Incision and drainage;
explore loculi

Tender swelling in natal cleft

Overlying erythema
May point and discharge
with protruding hair

Rectal examination is normal

Patient often
hirsute and sweaty

PILONIDAL ABSCESS
Incision and drainage,
leaving wound open to granulate

Ulcerated anal or
perianal mass

Biopsy

Squamous cell
carcinoma

ANAL CARCINOMA
Radiotherapy,
chemotherapy

Operation
if failure of above

The following is a discussion of the treatment of some of the conditions presented in Chapters 1, 2, 6, 7 and 8.

STOMAS

Intestinal stomas may be constructed from the ileum (ileostomy) or colon (colostomy) and brought to the skin either as a single end or as an intact loop with a side opening (usually for temporary diversion of the faecal stream). A stoma is a neoanus, constructed when the anus itself has been removed or when diversion of the faecal stream from the distal bowel is desirable, such as in emergency left-sided colonic surgery where there is a need to 'rest' distal diseased bowel or protect an anastomosis.

INFLAMMATORY BOWEL DISEASE

Crohn's disease may affect the whole bowel from mouth to anus, whereas ulcerative colitis is primarily a large bowel disease. Both conditions may relapse and remit with variable frequency and may be associated with a range of systemic manifestations including arthritides, erythema nodosum and iritis. Ulcerative colitis, when affecting the whole colon, is a premalignant condition and the risk is proportional to the length of the history.

Patients presenting with uncomplicated proctitis are treated primarily with topical steroids by suppository or enema. The very ill patient with pancolitis may require intravenous high-dose steroids, with rectal steroid enemas in addition. Metronidazole is given to treat infection and has a specific therapeutic effect in Crohn's disease. Mesalazine and sulphasalazine are used to maintain remission, particularly in ulcerative colitis, and azathioprine may also be used.

The indications for operation are elective and emergency. Emergency surgery is undertaken for the acute illness of toxic megacolon in ulcerative colitis where the risk is perforation, or for peritonitis resulting from perforation. Elective operation is undertaken for the failure of medical treatment resulting in debilitating symptoms, for uncontrolled systemic illness and for dysplasia and impending malignancy.

Elective or emergency panproctocolectomy are common operations undertaken for ulcerative colitis. End ileostomy may be avoided by the construction of an ileal pouch with a pouch–anal anastomosis, either with a covering ileostomy or as a single-stage procedure. Operations undertaken for Crohn's disease reflect the segmental distribution of the diseased bowel.

COLORECTAL CANCER

Operation is the treatment of choice both for palliation and cure. Palliative surgery is undertaken for unresectable disease where there is local invasion to unresectable or vital structures, or where there are distant unresectable metastases.

Curative procedures aim to remove the primary tumour and the associated mesenteric lymph nodes. Intestinal continuity is restored if this is consistent with cure. Operations include right hemicolectomy, transverse colectomy, left hemicolectomy, sigmoid colectomy, anterior resection (the upper/middle third of the rectum is excised with a primary anastomosis), and abdominoperineal excision of the rectum (the rectum and anal canal are excised and the bowel is brought to skin as an end colostomy). For left-sided colonic emergencies, a Hartmann's operation consists of colonic and/or rectal excision, oversewing of the rectal stump and end sigmoid colostomy. Colorectal continuity may be restored later.

Successful anastomosis should be tension-free in well-prepared bowel. For emergency surgery with unprepared bowel, obstruction or peritonitis a defunctioning intestinal stoma is usually raised, or both bowel ends are brought to the skin.

INTRODUCTION

Swellings in these areas are common. They account for about one in ten of outpatient presentations and are therefore frequently found in finals examinations.

The majority of lumps in these areas are hernias. A hernia is a protrusion of a viscus or part of a viscus through an abnormal opening in the walls of its containing cavity. It usually has three components: the sac, the coverings of the sac and the contents of the sac.

Hernias may be:

a. reducible
b. irreducible
c. obstructed
d. strangulated

An irreducible hernia is said to be obstructed if intestinal obstruction complicates the hernia. The term is not commonly used. If the blood supply to the hernia is compromised (implying impending gangrene and perforation) then the hernia is said to be strangulated.

9. LUMPS IN THE GROIN AND SCROTUM

9.1 LUMP IN GROIN

Locate the lump anatomically

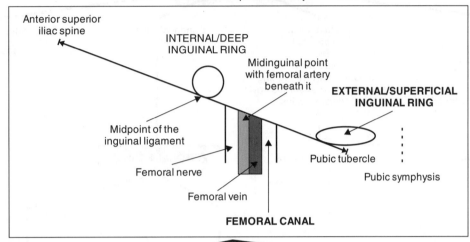

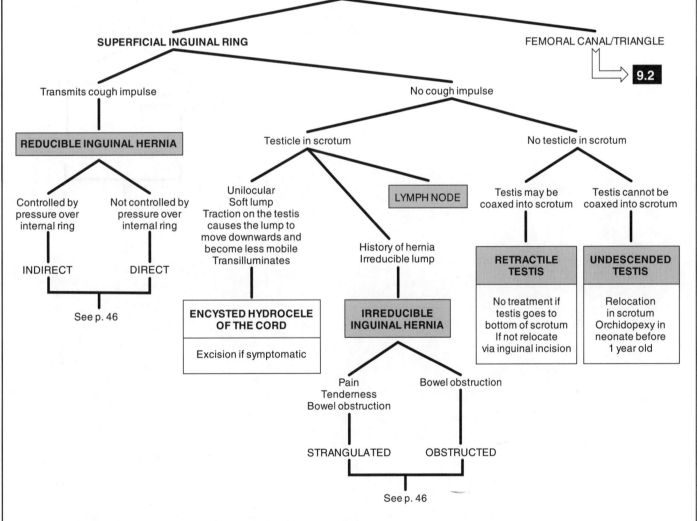

SUPERFICIAL INGUINAL RING

FEMORAL CANAL/TRIANGLE → **9.2**

Transmits cough impulse

No cough impulse

REDUCIBLE INGUINAL HERNIA

Testicle in scrotum

No testicle in scrotum

Controlled by pressure over internal ring — **INDIRECT**

Not controlled by pressure over internal ring — **DIRECT**

See p. 46

Unilocular
Soft lump
Traction on the testis causes the lump to move downwards and become less mobile
Transilluminates

LYMPH NODE

History of hernia
Irreducible lump

Testis may be coaxed into scrotum

Testis cannot be coaxed into scrotum

ENCYSTED HYDROCELE OF THE CORD

Excision if symptomatic

IRREDUCIBLE INGUINAL HERNIA

Pain
Tenderness
Bowel obstruction

Bowel obstruction

STRANGULATED

OBSTRUCTED

See p. 46

RETRACTILE TESTIS

No treatment if testis goes to bottom of scrotum
If not relocate via inguinal incision

UNDESCENDED TESTIS

Relocation in scrotum
Orchidopexy in neonate before 1 year old

9.2 LUMP IN FEMORAL CANAL/TRIANGLE

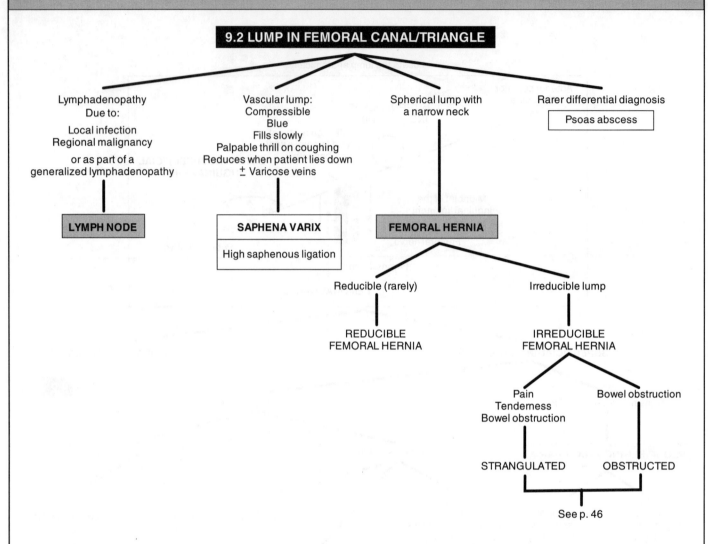

Lymphadenopathy
Due to:

Local infection
Regional malignancy

or as part of a
generalized lymphadenopathy

LYMPH NODE

Vascular lump:
Compressible
Blue
Fills slowly
Palpable thrill on coughing
Reduces when patient lies down
± Varicose veins

SAPHENA VARIX

High saphenous ligation

Spherical lump with
a narrow neck

FEMORAL HERNIA

Rarer differential diagnosis

Psoas abscess

Reducible (rarely)

REDUCIBLE
FEMORAL HERNIA

Irreducible lump

IRREDUCIBLE
FEMORAL HERNIA

Pain
Tenderness
Bowel obstruction

Bowel obstruction

STRANGULATED

OBSTRUCTED

See p. 46

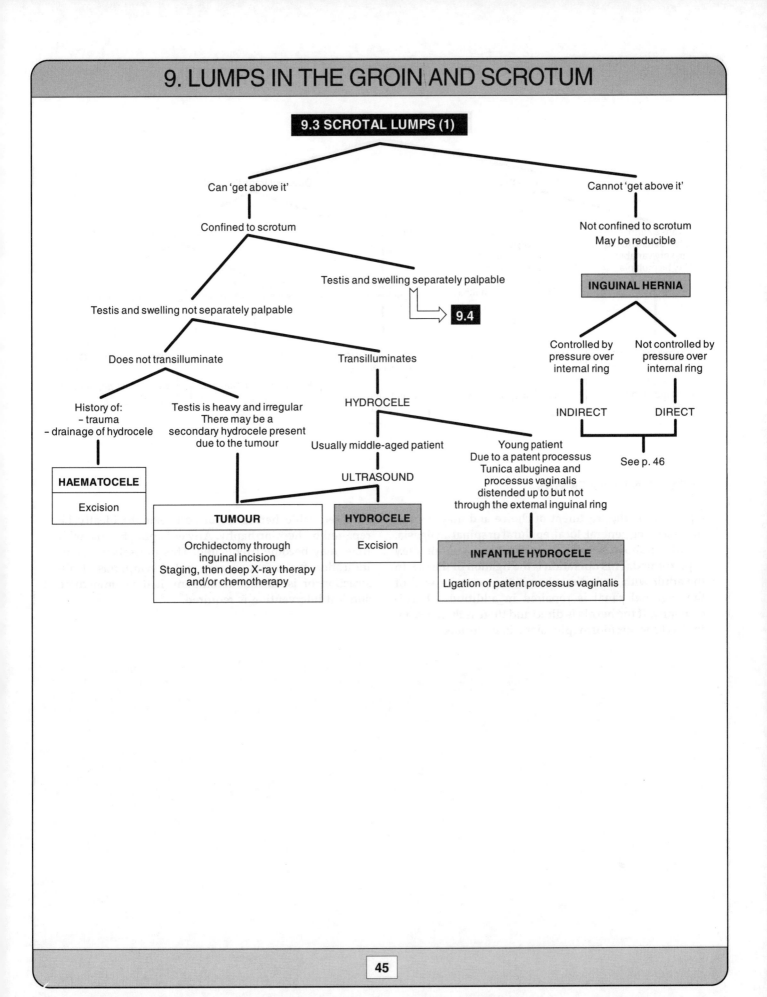

9.3 SCROTAL LUMPS (1)

Can 'get above it'

Confined to scrotum

Testis and swelling separately palpable → **9.4**

Testis and swelling not separately palpable

Does not transilluminate

History of:
– trauma
– drainage of hydrocele

HAEMATOCELE

Excision

Testis is heavy and irregular
There may be a secondary hydrocele present due to the tumour

TUMOUR

Orchidectomy through inguinal incision
Staging, then deep X-ray therapy and/or chemotherapy

Transilluminates

HYDROCELE

Usually middle-aged patient

ULTRASOUND

HYDROCELE

Excision

Young patient
Due to a patent processus
Tunica albuginea and processus vaginalis distended up to but not through the external inguinal ring

INFANTILE HYDROCELE

Ligation of patent processus vaginalis

Cannot 'get above it'

Not confined to scrotum
May be reducible

INGUINAL HERNIA

Controlled by pressure over internal ring

Not controlled by pressure over internal ring

INDIRECT

DIRECT

See p. 46

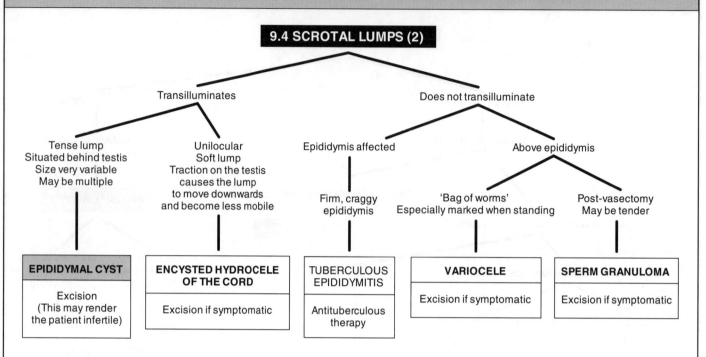

TREATMENT OF HERNIAS

Operation is the treatment of choice and may be performed using general, local, epidural or spinal analgesia.

All childhood hernias are indirect and a herniotomy is performed. This operation is the ligation of the sac. In the adult with an indirect hernia the posterior wall of the inguinal canal is repaired in addition – herniorrhaphy. If the hernia is direct and there is therefore no indirect sac, herniorrhaphy alone is performed.

A reducible hernia in an adult should ideally be repaired by herniorrhaphy. Any enlarging hernia, with time, may become irreducible. This in itself is not an indication for urgent surgery, but if symptoms of obstruction or ischaemia accompany it then immediate surgical intervention is required.

INTRODUCTION

Breast problems account for 15–20% of new surgical outpatient referrals. The majority of these patients present with a lump in the breast and may fear than they have cancer.

In approximately 20% of such women subsequent investigation will reveal a cancer which now affects 1 in 14. It is thus imperative to understand how to assess and manage breast cancer presentations.

Breast screening

There is evidence (widely but not universally accepted) that mammography every 2–3 years in patients of 50–75 years reduces the mortality from breast cancer. This is the basis for the screening programmes now offered to all females in the UK. This has led to a large increase in the number of premalignant and early malignant tumours being treated by minimal surgery and meticulous follow-up. The 'right' treatment for screening detected disease is still not clear and many of these patients are therefore entered into clinical trials.

Mammography

The prime role of mammography in screening or follow-up is to detect cancer in asymptomatic and high risk individuals (age, past history, family history). Signs of carcinoma on mammography include calcified or thickened breast tissue, which may then be localised and excised. It is also increasingly being used as a diagnostic tool, but beware the false negative mammogram. In general palpable lumps which are not cysts are removed to get histological material.

10. LUMPS IN THE BREAST

10.1 INITIAL ASSESSMENT

HISTORY

30–50 years old	18–35 years old	40+ years old
Cyclical pain	Painless	Painless
Past history of cysts or	May be multiple	Positive family history
excision of benign lumps	May be past history	Commoner in multiparous
		who haven't breast-fed

EXAMINATION

Smooth, rounded outline (not fluctuant)
Ill-defined areas of thickening – especially upper outer quadrant

Usually smooth, may be lobulated if large
Highly mobile around breast
'Breast mouse'
Usually less than 1 cm

Hard, ill-defined margin
Tethered to skin
Skin dimpling

Nipple inversion
Bloodstained discharge
Axillary lymphadenopathy

Peau d'orange
Fixed to pectoralis major or skin
Ulceration

Hepatosplenomegaly
Weight loss and cachexia

Rarer differential diagnoses
- Breast abscess
- Cystosarcoma phylloides
- Giant fibroadenoma

Probably
BENIGN MAMMARY DYSPLASIA

Probably
FIBROADENOMA

Probably
CARCINOMA

Attempt FINE NEEDLE ASPIRATION

Fluid recovered

No fluid recovered
Therefore residual lump
Cellular aspirate analysed

Fluid not bloodstained
Lump disappears and does not recur more than once
Cytology negative

Bloodstained fluid or residual lump

Cytology

**CYST OF
BENIGN MAMMARY DYSPLASIA**

No further treatment

CYTOLOGY NEGATIVE

CYTOLOGY POSITIVE

Excision biopsy

BENIGN

Discharged

MALIGNANT

Staging: Chest X-ray
± Liver function tests
± Ultrasound of liver
± Bone scan

→ **10.2**

10.2 MALIGNANT BREAST DISEASE (1)

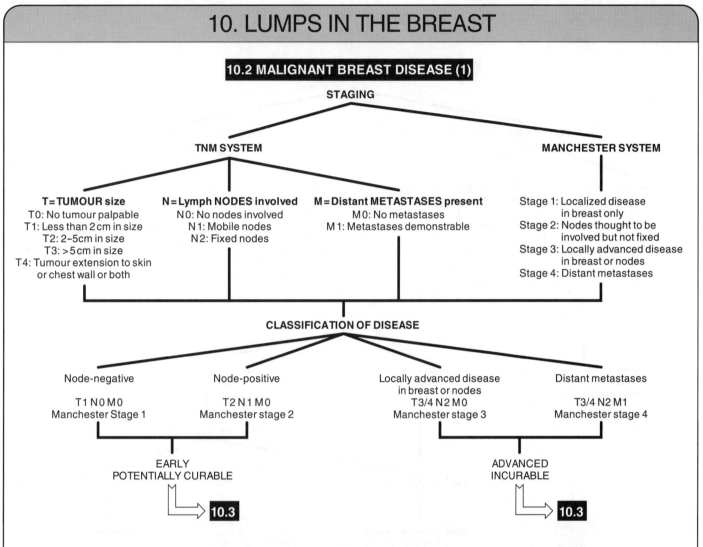

STAGING

TNM SYSTEM

MANCHESTER SYSTEM

T=TUMOUR size
T0: No tumour palpable
T1: Less than 2 cm in size
T2: 2–5 cm in size
T3: >5 cm in size
T4: Tumour extension to skin
or chest wall or both

N=Lymph NODES involved
N0: No nodes involved
N1: Mobile nodes
N2: Fixed nodes

M=Distant METASTASES present
M0: No metastases
M1: Metastases demonstrable

Stage 1: Localized disease
in breast only
Stage 2: Nodes thought to be
involved but not fixed
Stage 3: Locally advanced disease
in breast or nodes
Stage 4: Distant metastases

CLASSIFICATION OF DISEASE

Node-negative

T1 N0 M0
Manchester Stage 1

Node-positive

T2 N1 M0
Manchester stage 2

Locally advanced disease
in breast or nodes
T3/4 N2 M0
Manchester stage 3

Distant metastases

T3/4 N2 M1
Manchester stage 4

EARLY
POTENTIALLY CURABLE

→ **10.3**

ADVANCED
INCURABLE

→ **10.3**

There are many staging systems of breast cancer, each with many versions (at least 27 versions of TNM)
Remember the main categories:
'Early' disease – either node-positive or node-negative
'Advanced' disease – either locally advanced or metastatic

10.3 MALIGNANT BREAST DISEASE (2)

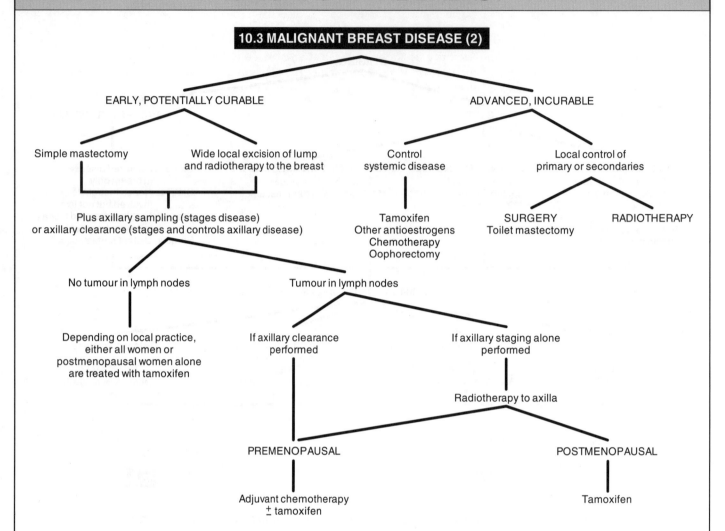

TREATMENT FACTS

1. Survival is independent of exact primary treatment: e.g. radical mastectomy – local excision and radiotherapy – simple mastectomy and radiotherapy
2. a. Locoregional recurrence (i.e. chest wall and axilla) is equally well controlled by radical surgery (axillary clearance) or conservative surgery with radiotherapy
    b. Conservative operation without radiotherapy leads to an unacceptable rate of local recurrence
    c. Radiotherapy does not prolong survival

3. Adjuvant chemotherapy is the only treatment shown to prolong survival in premenopausal node positive patients
4. Hormonal therapy prolongs survival in postmenopausal curable breast cancer

Note that local therapy may differ in certain centres, more aggressive surgery being the option for high-grade malignancy – e.g. some surgeons may proceed to mastectomy in node-negative disease for inflammatory or extensive intraductal carcinoma of the breast.

11. LUMPS IN THE SKIN

Skin lesions in the United Kingdom account for 13–18% of outpatient surgical referrals. The majority of these cause no great concern, but malignant lesions of the skin are increasing in incidence and therefore an accurate knowledge of the various guises of skin neoplasia is essential. Many types of skin lesion may ulcerate and these are discussed in Chapter 12.

This chapter should also be read in conjunction with Chapters 9, 10 and 13.

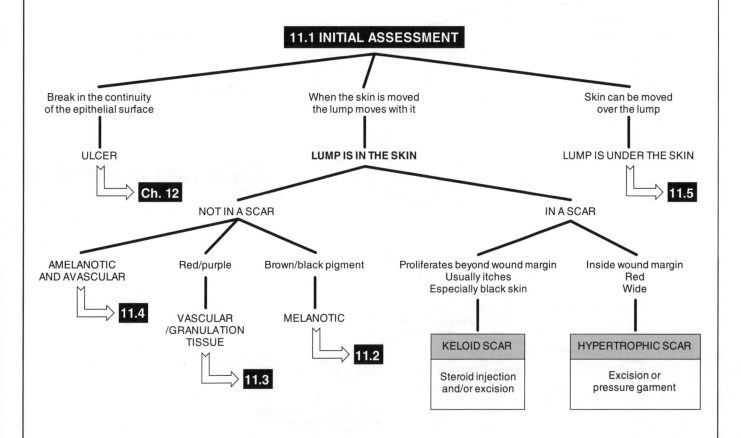

11. LUMPS IN THE SKIN

11.2 LUMP IN SKIN (1)

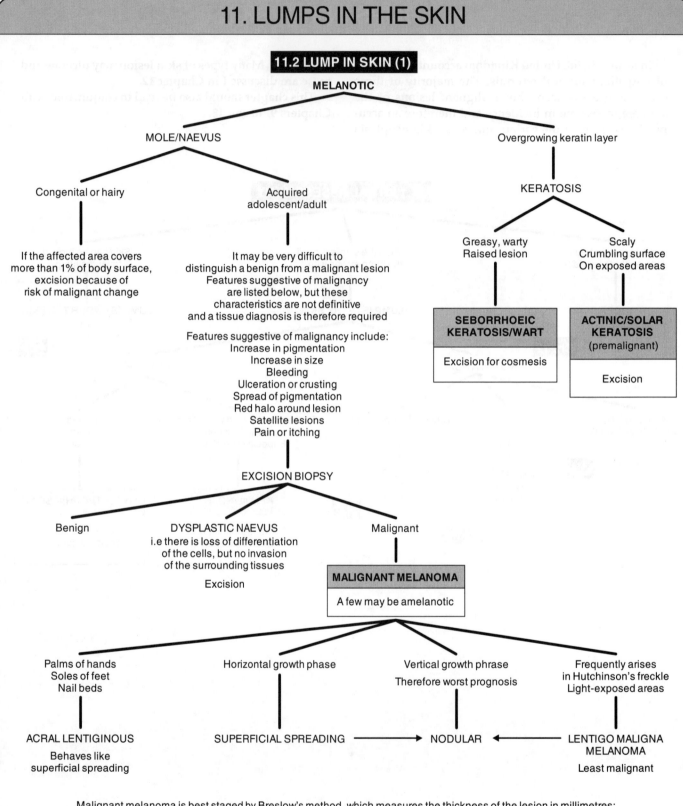

MELANOTIC

MOLE/NAEVUS

Overgrowing keratin layer

Congenital or hairy

If the affected area covers
more than 1% of body surface,
excision because of
risk of malignant change

**Acquired
adolescent/adult**

It may be very difficult to
distinguish a benign from a malignant lesion
Features suggestive of malignancy
are listed below, but these
characteristics are not definitive
and a tissue diagnosis is therefore required

Features suggestive of malignancy include:
Increase in pigmentation
Increase in size
Bleeding
Ulceration or crusting
Spread of pigmentation
Red halo around lesion
Satellite lesions
Pain or itching

EXCISION BIOPSY

Benign

DYSPLASTIC NAEVUS
i.e there is loss of differentiation
of the cells, but no invasion
of the surrounding tissues

Excision

Malignant

MALIGNANT MELANOMA

A few may be amelanotic

KERATOSIS

Greasy, warty
Raised lesion

**SEBORRHOEIC
KERATOSIS/WART**

Excision for cosmesis

Scaly
Crumbling surface
On exposed areas

**ACTINIC/SOLAR
KERATOSIS**
(premalignant)

Excision

Palms of hands
Soles of feet
Nail beds

ACRAL LENTIGINOUS

Behaves like
superficial spreading

Horizontal growth phase

SUPERFICIAL SPREADING →

Vertical growth phrase

Therefore worst prognosis

NODULAR ←

Frequently arises
in Hutchinson's freckle
Light-exposed areas

**LENTIGO MALIGNA
MELANOMA**

Least malignant

Malignant melanoma is best staged by Breslow's method, which measures the thickness of the lesion in millimetres:
the thicker the lesion the worse the prognosis and the wider the resection should be
Excision with a margin of normal tissue (of variable size) ± lymph node dissection is the normal treatment
Chemotherapy is for palliation only
Immunotherapy (interleukin-2) may have a role

11.3 LUMP IN SKIN (2)

VASCULAR/GRANULATION TISSUE

Raised

Slightly elevated/flat

Soft/compressible

Hard

Painful

Painless

Young people
Soft
Compressible

Rounded
Granulation tissue
Bleeds frequently

History of
penetrating injury

Multifocal
Bluish-red

1–3 mm
Under nail

STRAWBERRY NAEVUS

Leave it as most will eventually disappear

PYOGENIC GRANULOMA

Excision

KAPOSI'S SARCOMA

Consider HIV status and appropriate work-up

Single lesions are excised
Radiotherapy for multiple sites

GLOMUS TUMOUR

Excision

2–3 mm
Multiple
Bright red spots

Especially on face, neck and scalp
Present from birth
Asymmetrical outline

Central arteriole serving capillaries

CAMPBELL DE MORGAN SPOTS

Leave them

PORT WINE STAIN

Laser for cosmetic defect

SPIDER NAEVUS or TELANGIECTASIA

Seen in:

– liver disease
– hereditary haemorrhagic telangiectasia

Up to five may be normal

Usually no treatment required
If necessary, electrodesiccation

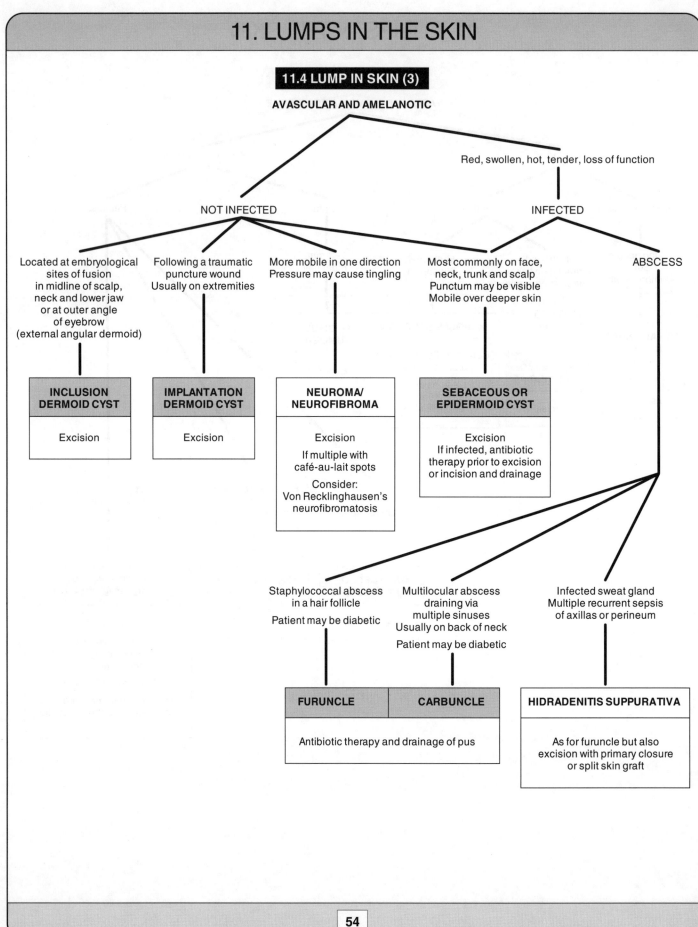

11.4 LUMP IN SKIN (3)

AVASCULAR AND AMELANOTIC

Red, swollen, hot, tender, loss of function

NOT INFECTED

INFECTED

Located at embryological sites of fusion in midline of scalp, neck and lower jaw or at outer angle of eyebrow (external angular dermoid)

Following a traumatic puncture wound Usually on extremities

More mobile in one direction Pressure may cause tingling

Most commonly on face, neck, trunk and scalp Punctum may be visible Mobile over deeper skin

ABSCESS

INCLUSION DERMOID CYST

Excision

IMPLANTATION DERMOID CYST

Excision

NEUROMA/ NEUROFIBROMA

Excision

If multiple with café-au-lait spots

Consider: Von Recklinghausen's neurofibromatosis

SEBACEOUS OR EPIDERMOID CYST

Excision If infected, antibiotic therapy prior to excision or incision and drainage

Staphylococcal abscess in a hair follicle

Patient may be diabetic

Multilocular abscess draining via multiple sinuses Usually on back of neck

Patient may be diabetic

Infected sweat gland Multiple recurrent sepsis of axillas or perineum

FURUNCLE	**CARBUNCLE**
Antibiotic therapy and drainage of pus	

HIDRADENITIS SUPPURATIVA

As for furuncle but also excision with primary closure or split skin graft

11. LUMPS IN THE SKIN

11.5 LUMP UNDER THE SKIN

PULSATILE

Machine-like murmur
on auscultation
Collapsing pulse distal to it

ARTERIOVENOUS MALFORMATION

Excision

May be a history of surgery
(especially vascular or trauma)

ANEURYSM

Excision or grafting

Non-pulsatile

In some instances the diagnosis of these lumps
depends on their anatomical location,
e.g. Lumps in groin or scrotum see Chapter 9
Lumps in the neck see Chapter 24

Any subcutaneous tissues or structures
may form benign or malignant tumours
Most of these that present as lumps in the skin
require histology to make the diagnosis;
a few, however (listed separately below) are characteristic
If a soft tissue malignant tumour is suspected,
an incision biopsy is taken via a small, carefully placed incision
that is unlikely to compromise subsequent definitive surgery

Rarer differential diagnoses
requiring histology for diagnosis, e.g.

Angioma
Fibroma
Neuroma
Angiosarcoma
Rhabdomyosarcoma
Fibrosarcoma
Osteosarcoma
Chondrosarcoma

Dorsum of the wrist, hand
and around the ankle

Hemispherical
Hard, fluctuant consistency
Weakly transilluminable

GANGLION

Excision

Can present anywhere

Lobulated/soft

LIPOMA

Excision if inconvenient or unsightly

If multiple and painful

MULTIPLE LIPOMATOSIS/ DERCUM'S DISEASE

Can rarely undergo
malignant change

LIPOSARCOMA

12. ULCERS

An ulcer is a break in the continuity of an epithelial surface

12.1 CLINICAL FEATURES

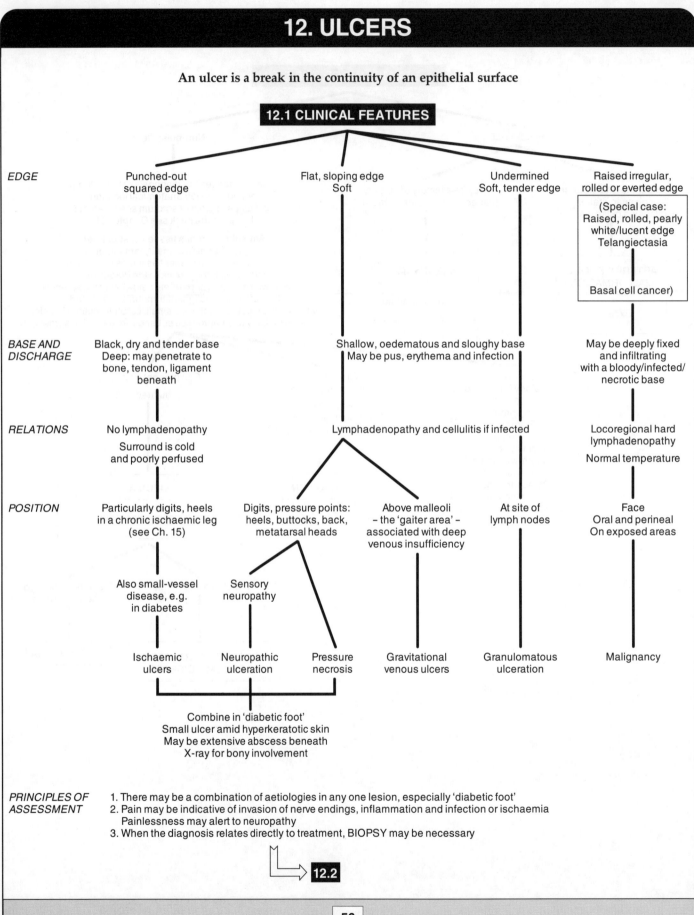

EDGE	Punched-out squared edge	Flat, sloping edge Soft	Undermined Soft, tender edge	Raised irregular, rolled or everted edge

(Special case: Raised, rolled, pearly white/lucent edge Telangiectasia

Basal cell cancer)

BASE AND DISCHARGE	Black, dry and tender base Deep: may penetrate to bone, tendon, ligament beneath	Shallow, oedematous and sloughy base May be pus, erythema and infection	May be deeply fixed and infiltrating with a bloody/infected/ necrotic base
RELATIONS	No lymphadenopathy Surround is cold and poorly perfused	Lymphadenopathy and cellulitis if infected	Locoregional hard lymphadenopathy Normal temperature
POSITION	Particularly digits, heels in a chronic ischaemic leg (see Ch. 15)	Digits, pressure points: heels, buttocks, back, metatarsal heads / Above malleoli – the 'gaiter area' – associated with deep venous insufficiency	At site of lymph nodes / Face Oral and perineal On exposed areas

Also small-vessel disease, e.g. in diabetes

Sensory neuropathy

Ischaemic ulcers	Neuropathic ulceration	Pressure necrosis	Gravitational venous ulcers	Granulomatous ulceration	Malignancy

Combine in 'diabetic foot'
Small ulcer amid hyperkeratotic skin
May be extensive abscess beneath
X-ray for bony involvement

PRINCIPLES OF ASSESSMENT
1. There may be a combination of aetiologies in any one lesion, especially 'diabetic foot'
2. Pain may be indicative of invasion of nerve endings, inflammation and infection or ischaemia
   Painlessness may alert to neuropathy
3. When the diagnosis relates directly to treatment, BIOPSY may be necessary

12.2

12. ULCERS

12.2 FURTHER INVESTIGATION (1)

Ischaemic arterial ulcers → **12.3**

Venous (gravitational) ulcers → **12.3**

Suspect
- Malignancy
- Granulomatous ulceration

BIOPSY
Small lesions may be diagnosed by excision biopsy

PRESSURE NECROSIS

Conservative care:

2-hourly turning for relief of direct and shearing forces

Prevention of infection and control of diabetes

Optimum nutritional intake; control of obesity

Heals

Fails to heal

Plastic surgical reconstruction

Malignancy

Granuloma

TUBERCULOSIS SYPHILITIC ULCER

Antituberculous or antisyphilitic drug therapy as necessary

Painless raised, rolled edge (and see special case in Fig. 12.1)

Slow-growing May erode deeply

Areas exposed to ultraviolet light, e.g. on face and neck

BASAL CELL CARCINOMA

Excision biopsy/ deep curettage and local radiotherapy

Mole/naevus Usually pigmented

Clinical features of malignant melanoma (see Fig. 11.2)

Areas exposed to ultraviolet light, e.g. on face and neck

MALIGNANT MELANOMA

A minority are amelanotic

→ **11.2**

Painful/painless bleed and discharge Many sites Everted irregular and indurated edge

May arise in areas of chronic inflammation

Areas exposed to ultraviolet light, e.g. on face and neck

SQUAMOUS CELL CARCINOMA

Excision with a 1 cm margin Block dissection of regional nodes Radiosensitive Good prognosis

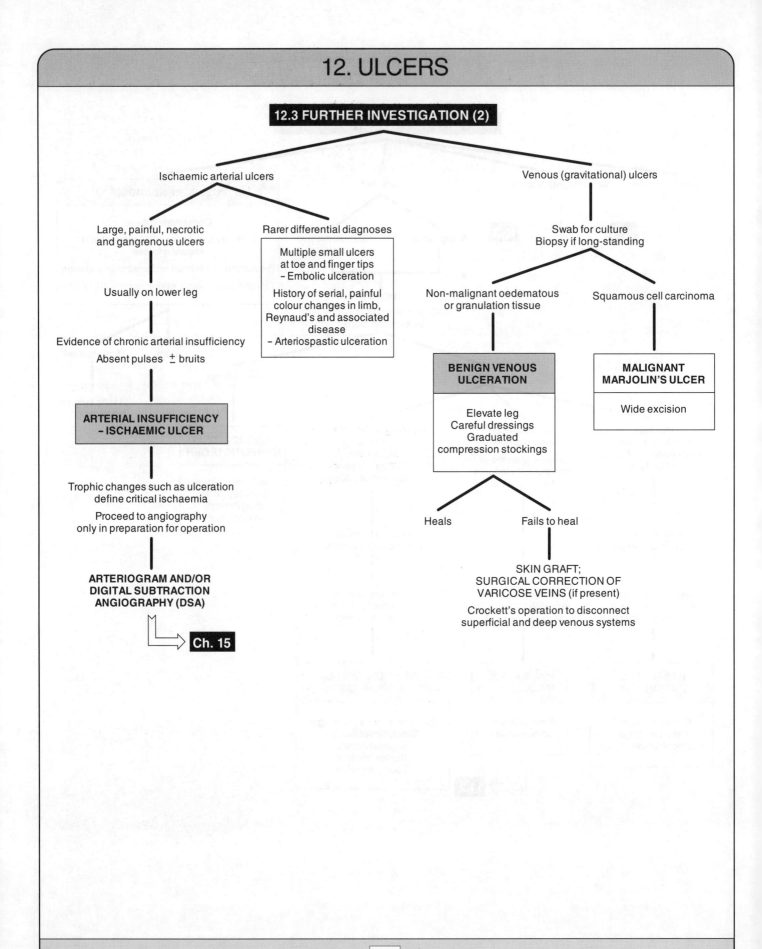

12.3 FURTHER INVESTIGATION (2)

Ischaemic arterial ulcers

Large, painful, necrotic and gangrenous ulcers

Usually on lower leg

Evidence of chronic arterial insufficiency
Absent pulses ± bruits

ARTERIAL INSUFFICIENCY – ISCHAEMIC ULCER

Trophic changes such as ulceration define critical ischaemia
Proceed to angiography only in preparation for operation

ARTERIOGRAM AND/OR DIGITAL SUBTRACTION ANGIOGRAPHY (DSA)

Ch. 15

Rarer differential diagnoses

Multiple small ulcers at toe and finger tips – Embolic ulceration

History of serial, painful colour changes in limb, Reynaud's and associated disease – Arteriospastic ulceration

Venous (gravitational) ulcers

Swab for culture
Biopsy if long-standing

Non-malignant oedematous or granulation tissue

Squamous cell carcinoma

BENIGN VENOUS ULCERATION

Elevate leg
Careful dressings
Graduated compression stockings

MALIGNANT MARJOLIN'S ULCER

Wide excision

Heals

Fails to heal

SKIN GRAFT;
SURGICAL CORRECTION OF VARICOSE VEINS (if present)

Crockett's operation to disconnect superficial and deep venous systems

13. LYMPHADENOPATHY

INTRODUCTION

Lymphadenopathy (enlarged, palpable nodes) is a common occurrence and can be either localised or generalized.

This division, although useful, can be misleading in two circumstances:

a. if there is only one clinically palpable chain of nodes in a patient with generalized lymphadenopathy

b. in certain disorders that can cause both a localized and a generalized lymphadenopathy.

The aim of this chapter is to remind you of the major routes of lymphatic drainage and common causes of lymphadenopathy. It is very important to take detailed histories, as this will yield the diagnosis in the majority of cases.

The possible causes include:

Localized

a. Infections:
   - (i) Bacterial – e.g. otitis media, pharyngitis, tuberculosis
   - (ii) Fungal – e.g. actinomycosis
   - (iii) Viral – e.g. cat scratch fever, lymphogranuloma venereum

b. Malignancy:
   - (i) Primary – Hodgkin's and non-Hodgkin's lymphoma
   - (ii) Secondary

Generalized

a. Infections:
   - (i) Bacterial – e.g. brucellosis, syphilis, tuberculosis, endocarditis
   - (ii) Fungal – e.g. histoplasmosis
   - (iii) Viral – e.g. infectious mononucleosis, measles, rubella, viral hepatitis
   - (iv) Protozoal – e.g. toxoplasmosis

b. Malignancy:
   - (i) Primary – Hodgkin's and non-Hodgkin's lymphoma, chronic lymphocytic leukaemia, acute lymphocytic leukaemia
   - (ii) Secondary

c. Non-infectious inflammatory diseases – e.g. sarcoidosis, rheumatoid arthritis, systemic lupus erythematosus

d. Others: – e.g. drug reactions, angioimmunoblastic lymphadenopathy, hyperthyroidism

13. LYMPHADENOPATHY

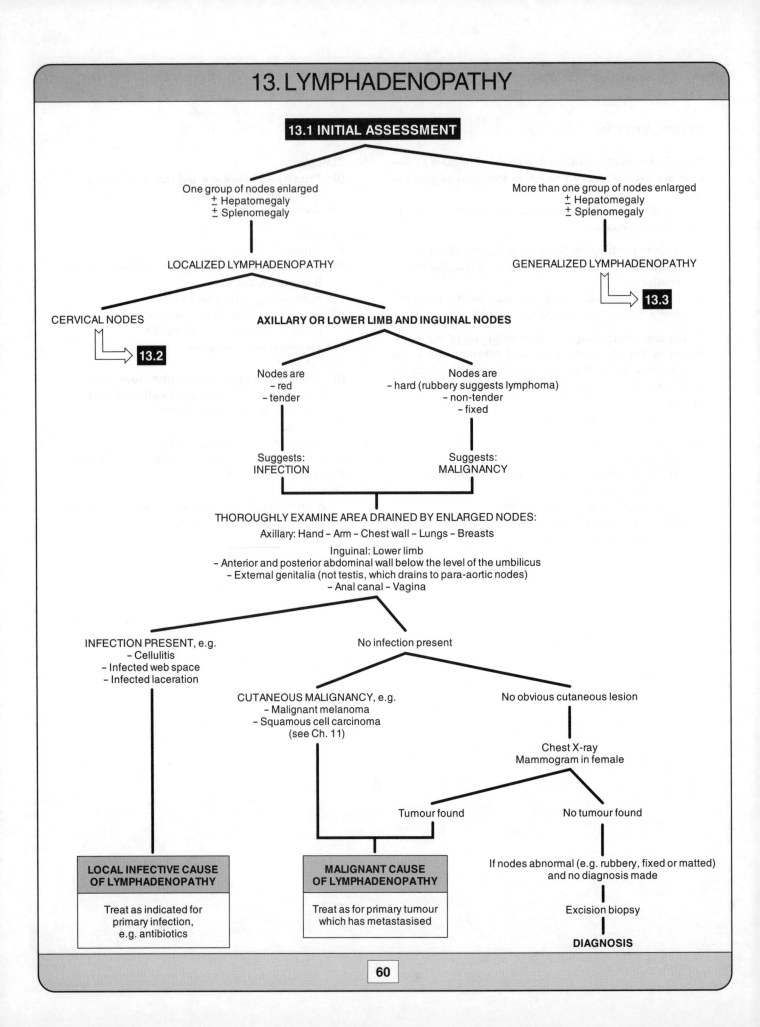

13.1 INITIAL ASSESSMENT

One group of nodes enlarged
± Hepatomegaly
± Splenomegaly

More than one group of nodes enlarged
± Hepatomegaly
± Splenomegaly

LOCALIZED LYMPHADENOPATHY

GENERALIZED LYMPHADENOPATHY → 13.3

CERVICAL NODES → 13.2

AXILLARY OR LOWER LIMB AND INGUINAL NODES

Nodes are
– red
– tender

Nodes are
– hard (rubbery suggests lymphoma)
– non-tender
– fixed

Suggests:
INFECTION

Suggests:
MALIGNANCY

THOROUGHLY EXAMINE AREA DRAINED BY ENLARGED NODES:

Axillary: Hand – Arm – Chest wall – Lungs – Breasts

Inguinal: Lower limb
– Anterior and posterior abdominal wall below the level of the umbilicus
– External genitalia (not testis, which drains to para-aortic nodes)
– Anal canal – Vagina

INFECTION PRESENT, e.g.
– Cellulitis
– Infected web space
– Infected laceration

No infection present

CUTANEOUS MALIGNANCY, e.g.
– Malignant melanoma
– Squamous cell carcinoma
(see Ch. 11)

No obvious cutaneous lesion

Chest X-ray
Mammogram in female

Tumour found

No tumour found

If nodes abnormal (e.g. rubbery, fixed or matted)
and no diagnosis made

Excision biopsy

DIAGNOSIS

**LOCAL INFECTIVE CAUSE
OF LYMPHADENOPATHY**

Treat as indicated for
primary infection,
e.g. antibiotics

**MALIGNANT CAUSE
OF LYMPHADENOPATHY**

Treat as for primary tumour
which has metastasised

13. LYMPHADENOPATHY

13.2 LOCALIZED LYMPHADENOPATHY IN CERVICAL NODES

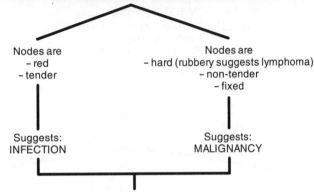

Nodes are
 – red
 – tender

Nodes are
– hard (rubbery suggests lymphoma)
 – non-tender
 – fixed

Suggests:
INFECTION

Suggests:
MALIGNANCY

THOROUGHLY EXAMINE AREA DRAINED BY ENLARGED NODES:
– Scalp – Nose and paranasal space – Mouth and tongue
– Neck – Pharynx and larynx

(It is important to ask an ENT surgeon to examine the larynx and nasopharynx before biopsy
since preliminary biopsy of nodes of laryngeal carcinoma prejudices the cure)

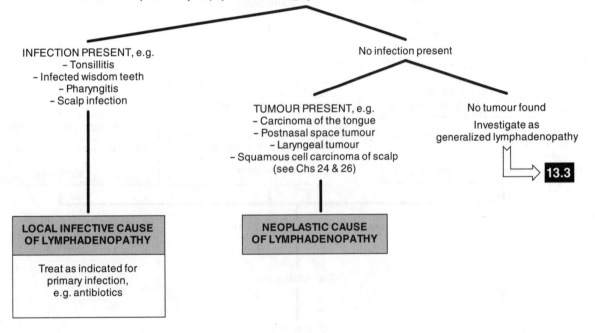

INFECTION PRESENT, e.g.
 – Tonsillitis
 – Infected wisdom teeth
 – Pharyngitis
 – Scalp infection

No infection present

TUMOUR PRESENT, e.g.
 – Carcinoma of the tongue
 – Postnasal space tumour
 – Laryngeal tumour
– Squamous cell carcinoma of scalp
 (see Chs 24 & 26)

No tumour found

Investigate as
generalized lymphadenopathy

13.3

**LOCAL INFECTIVE CAUSE
OF LYMPHADENOPATHY**

Treat as indicated for
primary infection,
e.g. antibiotics

**NEOPLASTIC CAUSE
OF LYMPHADENOPATHY**

13. LYMPHADENOPATHY

13.3 GENERALIZED LYMPHADENOPATHY

INVESTIGATIONS include:
Blood for: Full blood count + Differential
Film for microscopy
Paul–Bunnell monospot
HIV test – after counselling
Sabin–Feldman dye test
Angiotensin converting enzyme levels
Treponemal serology

Mantoux test
Chest X-ray
Ultrasound of liver, spleen and abdominal nodes

INFECTIOUS CAUSES

INVESTIGATION	DIAGNOSIS
Non-specific (VDRL-positive) Specific (VDRL-negative)	**TREPONEMAL DISEASE**
Positive Mantoux test	**TUBERCULOSIS**
Positive Paul–Bunnell test	**INFECTIOUS MONONUCLEOSIS**
Positive Sabin–Feldman dye test	**TOXOPLASMOSIS**
HIV-antibody-positive	**HIV INFECTION**

OTHERS

Elevated serum ACE levels

SARCOID

Rarer differential diagnoses include:

Non-infectious inflammatory diseases,
e.g. Rheumatoid arthritis
–Systemic lupus erythematosus

Angioimmunoblastic lymphadenopathy
Sinus histiocytosis and lymphadenopathy
Reaction to drugs, e.g. hydantoins
Secondary carcinoma
Hyperthyroidism

HAEMATOLOGICAL CAUSES
These will usually present with accompanying systemic symptoms:

Abnormal blood film
± Abnormal bone marrow biopsy
± Normochromic, normocytic anaemia
± Thrombocytopenia

ACUTE LYMPHOCYTIC LEUKAEMIA

CHRONIC LYMPHOCYTIC LEUKAEMIA

LYMPHOMA

Diagnosis still often depends on biopsy

Excision biopsy

DIAGNOSIS

INTRODUCTION

Pain in the legs is a common symptom and may relate to conditions requiring prompt management of a limb in peril. The common causes are considered below according to whether they are of sudden onset, with an acute presentation such as acute arterial occlusion and deep venous thrombosis, or have a more insidious presentation such as claudication. Leg pains resulting from trauma are not included within this section.

Case history

A 52-year-old smoker calls his general practitioner in a panic complaining of an excruciatingly painful, cold, 'dead' left leg. He is unable to move his foot and toes, which have also gone numb. The GP elicits a telephone history of symptoms lasting 30 minutes and, while reading through the patient's record, notes a previous medical history of myocardial infarction 4 years before and subsequent mitral valve replacement. The patient is noted to be taking digoxin and aspirin.

1. What does the GP do next, and what is his working diagnosis?

The GP rings the local hospital and warns the surgical registrar that he is bringing in an emergency with a probable acutely ischaemic limb. He visits the patient and on examination finds a cold limb with reduced power and sensation. There are no pulses below the left femoral pulse and there are no signs of abnormal circulation on the contralateral side. The patient is in atrial fibrillation and admits to not having taken any of his medication for some time. He is taken to hospital urgently.

2. The surgical registrar agrees with the clinical findings of the GP. What diagnosis does he make and what does he do next?

The diagnosis of acute arterial embolism is made. The surgeon takes the patient to theatre and evacuates the embolus from the left popliteal artery with a Fogarty catheter. On-table arteriography reveals a postoperative patent circulation distal to the embolic occlusion.

3. How would you further manage this patient?

14.1 INITIAL ASSESSMENT

Deep pain in thigh/calf compartment
or whole leg
→ **14.2**

Localized to skin,
soft tissues or veins

Pain in legs radiating from the back
Exacerbated by bending or particular movements
→ **15.3**

SIGNS OF INFLAMMATION

Tender area of skin
which is hyperaemic, warm and red

Thin, red tender streak
on the skin

Red and very tender
superficial vein

May be localized lymphadenopathy

May be paronychia or peripheral ulceration

Inguinal lymphadenopathy

History of local intravenous catheterization
or inflammation of varicose veins

Patient often has high fever

CELLULITIS
Antibiotics

LYMPHANGITIS
Antibiotics

SUPERFICIAL THROMBOPHLEBITIS

Multiple attacks with no local predisposing factors,
often in different areas, may be associated with
malignancy (especially pancreatic carcinoma)

THROMBOPHLEBITIS MIGRANS

14. ACUTE NON-TRAUMATIC LEG PAIN

14.2 DEEP PAIN IN THIGH/CALF COMPARTMENT

Pain and 'numbness' in limb
Paresis/paralysis
Paraesthesiae or hypoaesthesia

ON EXAMINATION

Pale, pulseless, cold limb
Mottled, dusky-coloured periphery with reduced sensation

May be evidence of embolic source, e.g. atrial fibrillation, cardiac dysrhythmias, aortic/mitral valve disease, aortic aneurysm, ischaemic heart disease, recent myocardial infarction

Suggests:

No evidence of embolic source

Generalized features of peripheral vascular disease, abnormal pulses and bruits

Suggests:

ACUTE ARTERIAL EMBOLISM	ACUTE ARTERIAL THROMBOSIS
Level of occlusion defined clinically by level below which pulses cannot be felt Urgent intervention necessary Cool limb to reduce metabolic requirement Care to avoid pressure necrosis	

Urgent FOGARTY CATHETER EMBOLECTOMY
Peroperative angiography to exclude chronic vascular disease and confirm patency of distal vessels postembolectomy

Urgent angiography to localize stenosis and assess for reconstruction

Pain and uniform swelling
No paresis or sensory loss

ON EXAMINATION

Warm, tense, tender limb
Low-grade pyrexia

Increased risk if female, obese, taking the oral contraceptive pill, recent operation, childbirth

History of previous venous thrombosis

History of chronic joint disease

Absence of risk factors for venous thrombosis

DEEP VENOUS THROMBOSIS

(diagnosis may be confirmed by contrast venography/flow ultrasonography)

Pelvic/soleal (parafemoral) veins (also axillary veins)

Anticoagulate with i.v. heparin, then warfarin

RUPTURED BAKER'S CYST
(pulsion diverticulum from arthritic knee)

15. CHRONIC LEG PAINS AND CLAUDICATION

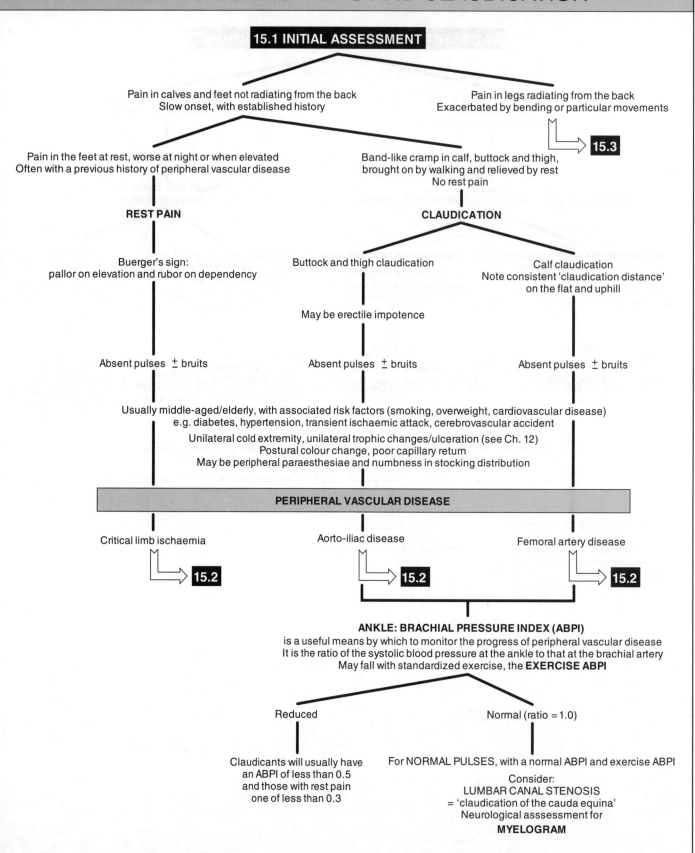

15.1 INITIAL ASSESSMENT

Pain in calves and feet not radiating from the back
Slow onset, with established history

Pain in legs radiating from the back
Exacerbated by bending or particular movements → **15.3**

Pain in the feet at rest, worse at night or when elevated
Often with a previous history of peripheral vascular disease

Band-like cramp in calf, buttock and thigh,
brought on by walking and relieved by rest
No rest pain

REST PAIN

CLAUDICATION

Buerger's sign:
pallor on elevation and rubor on dependency

Buttock and thigh claudication

Calf claudication
Note consistent 'claudication distance'
on the flat and uphill

May be erectile impotence

Absent pulses ± bruits

Absent pulses ± bruits

Absent pulses ± bruits

Usually middle-aged/elderly, with associated risk factors (smoking, overweight, cardiovascular disease)
e.g. diabetes, hypertension, transient ischaemic attack, cerebrovascular accident
Unilateral cold extremity, unilateral trophic changes/ulceration (see Ch. 12)
Postural colour change, poor capillary return
May be peripheral paraesthesiae and numbness in stocking distribution

PERIPHERAL VASCULAR DISEASE

Critical limb ischaemia → **15.2**

Aorto-iliac disease → **15.2**

Femoral artery disease → **15.2**

ANKLE: BRACHIAL PRESSURE INDEX (ABPI)
is a useful means by which to monitor the progress of peripheral vascular disease
It is the ratio of the systolic blood pressure at the ankle to that at the brachial artery
May fall with standardized exercise, the **EXERCISE ABPI**

Reduced

Normal (ratio = 1.0)

Claudicants will usually have
an ABPI of less than 0.5
and those with rest pain
one of less than 0.3

For NORMAL PULSES, with a normal ABPI and exercise ABPI

Consider:
LUMBAR CANAL STENOSIS
= 'claudication of the cauda equina'
Neurological asssessment for
MYELOGRAM

15.2 PERIPHERAL VASCULAR DISEASE

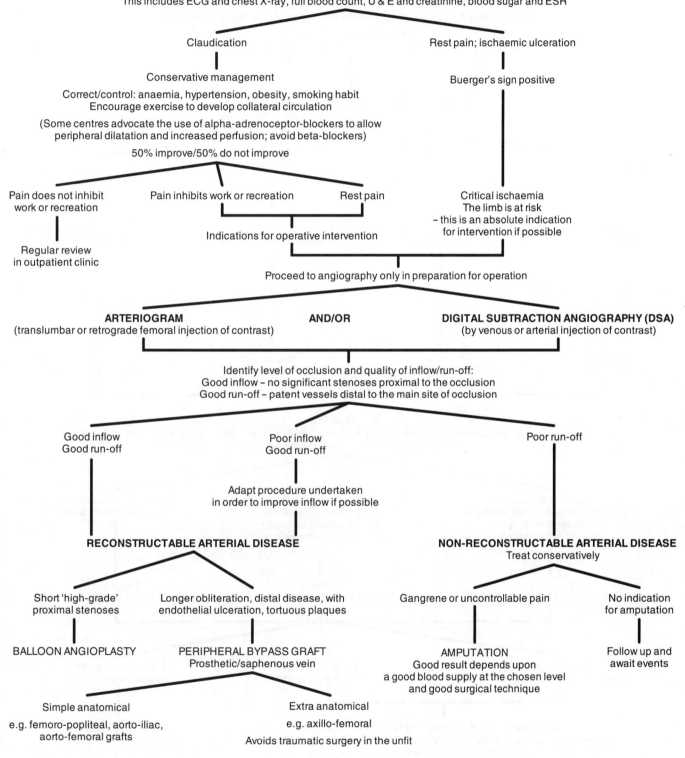

Work-up of these patients includes screening for risk factors and associated diseases
This includes ECG and chest X-ray, full blood count, U & E and creatinine, blood sugar and ESR

Claudication

Rest pain; ischaemic ulceration

Conservative management

Buerger's sign positive

Correct/control: anaemia, hypertension, obesity, smoking habit
Encourage exercise to develop collateral circulation

(Some centres advocate the use of alpha-adrenoceptor-blockers to allow
peripheral dilatation and increased perfusion; avoid beta-blockers)

50% improve/50% do not improve

Pain does not inhibit
work or recreation

Pain inhibits work or recreation

Rest pain

Critical ischaemia
The limb is at risk
– this is an absolute indication
for intervention if possible

Regular review
in outpatient clinic

Indications for operative intervention

Proceed to angiography only in preparation for operation

ARTERIOGRAM
(translumbar or retrograde femoral injection of contrast)

AND/OR

DIGITAL SUBTRACTION ANGIOGRAPHY (DSA)
(by venous or arterial injection of contrast)

Identify level of occlusion and quality of inflow/run-off:
Good inflow – no significant stenoses proximal to the occlusion
Good run-off – patent vessels distal to the main site of occlusion

Good inflow
Good run-off

Poor inflow
Good run-off

Poor run-off

Adapt procedure undertaken
in order to improve inflow if possible

RECONSTRUCTABLE ARTERIAL DISEASE

NON-RECONSTRUCTABLE ARTERIAL DISEASE
Treat conservatively

Short 'high-grade'
proximal stenoses

Longer obliteration, distal disease, with
endothelial ulceration, tortuous plaques

Gangrene or uncontrollable pain

No indication
for amputation

BALLOON ANGIOPLASTY

PERIPHERAL BYPASS GRAFT
Prosthetic/saphenous vein

AMPUTATION
Good result depends upon
a good blood supply at the chosen level
and good surgical technique

Follow up and
await events

Simple anatomical

e.g. femoro-popliteal, aorto-iliac,
aorto-femoral grafts

Extra anatomical

e.g. axillo-femoral

Avoids traumatic surgery in the unfit

15.3 LUMBOSACRAL NERVE ROOT COMPRESSION (1)

Pain in legs radiating from the back
Exacerbated by bending or particular movements

Straight-leg raising mimics the pain in the distribution of the affected nerve root

Tender lumbosacral spine
Concavity of spine on affected side with flexion of ipsilateral hip and knee

LUMBOSACRAL NERVE ROOT COMPRESSION

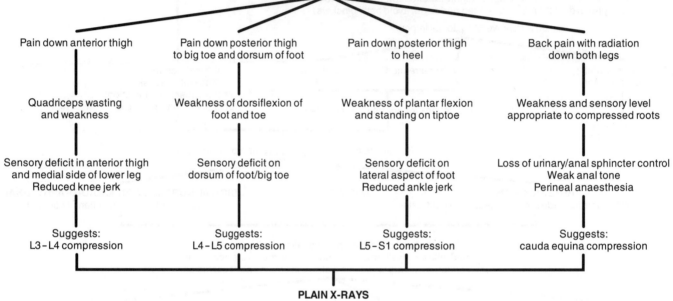

Pain down anterior thigh	Pain down posterior thigh to big toe and dorsum of foot	Pain down posterior thigh to heel	Back pain with radiation down both legs
Quadriceps wasting and weakness	Weakness of dorsiflexion of foot and toe	Weakness of plantar flexion and standing on tiptoe	Weakness and sensory level appropriate to compressed roots
Sensory deficit in anterior thigh and medial side of lower leg Reduced knee jerk	Sensory deficit on dorsum of foot/big toe	Sensory deficit on lateral aspect of foot Reduced ankle jerk	Loss of urinary/anal sphincter control Weak anal tone Perineal anaesthesia
Suggests: L3–L4 compression	Suggests: L4–L5 compression	Suggests: L5–S1 compression	Suggests: cauda equina compression

PLAIN X-RAYS
May indicate level of cord/root obstruction in conjunction with clinical picture,
and aid in interpreting myelograms; look for:

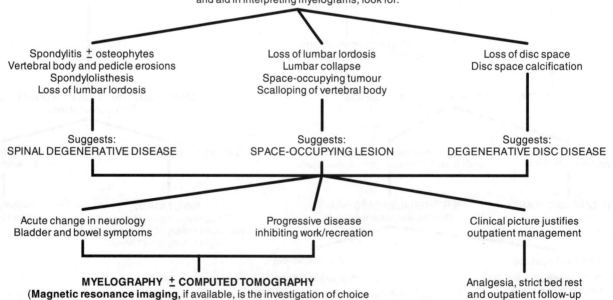

Spondylitis ± osteophytes Vertebral body and pedicle erosions Spondylolisthesis Loss of lumbar lordosis	Loss of lumbar lordosis Lumbar collapse Space-occupying tumour Scalloping of vertebral body	Loss of disc space Disc space calcification
Suggests: SPINAL DEGENERATIVE DISEASE	Suggests: SPACE-OCCUPYING LESION	Suggests: DEGENERATIVE DISC DISEASE

Acute change in neurology Bladder and bowel symptoms	Progressive disease inhibiting work/recreation	Clinical picture justifies outpatient management

MYELOGRAPHY ± COMPUTED TOMOGRAPHY
(**Magnetic resonance imaging,** if available, is the investigation of choice
for soft tissue disease)

Analgesia, strict bed rest
and outpatient follow-up

15.4 LUMBOSACRAL NERVE ROOT COMPRESSION (2)

MYELOGRAPHY ± COMPUTED TOMOGRAPHY
(**Magnetic resonance imaging,** if available, is the investigation of choice
for soft tissue disease)

Extradural mass
80%

METASTATIC TUMOUR

The commonest are lung, breast, prostate and kidney,
plus lymphoma and myeloma
Occur at multiple sites presenting as
bony collapse/space-occupying lesion

LUMBAR DISC PROLAPSE

Commonest at L4–L5 and L5–S1 levels with root compression
(rarely central disc prolapse causing cord compression)

The more lateral the disc protrusion the greater likelihood
of compression of the root above (consult a relevant diagram)

A free sequestrated fragment may affect > 1 level

OSTEOPHYTIC COMPRESSION

A common degenerative bony cause of spinal cord
or root compression

ABSCESS/TUBERCULOSIS

Most commonly *Staphylococcus aureus*;
local or haematogenous spread
Constitutional signs of infection
Risk of arteritis and infarction of cord
Meningitis if dura breached
Tuberculous spine usually presents as
vertebral collapse/disc erosion

HAEMATOMA

In the absence of injury, this is usually associated with
therapeutic anticoagulation

SPINAL DECOMPRESSION

e.g. DECOMPRESSIVE LAMINECTOMY and excision of
degenerative/infected/neoplastic tissue as necessary
± RADIOTHERAPY

HIGH-DOSE GLUCOCORTICOIDS
are used to reduce *acute* compression caused by oedema

Rarer differential diagnoses

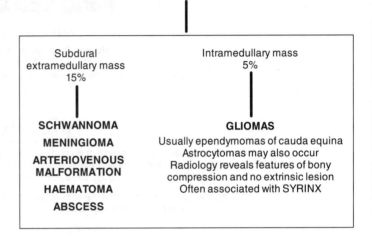

Subdural extramedullary mass
15%

SCHWANNOMA

MENINGIOMA

ARTERIOVENOUS MALFORMATION

HAEMATOMA

ABSCESS

Intramedullary mass
5%

GLIOMAS

Usually ependymomas of cauda equina
Astrocytomas may also occur
Radiology reveals features of bony
compression and no extrinsic lesion
Often associated with SYRINX

16. VARICOSE VEINS

The patient often compains of cosmetic disfigurement. Other symptoms include pain exacerbated by standing and relieved by elevation, and itching due to varicose eczema. Thrombophlebitis may occur in the varicose veins. Ulcers at the ankle are rare with simple varicose veins and are more usually associated with pathology in the deep veins (see Ch. 12). Thin-walled varicose veins may bleed spontaneously.

16.1 INITIAL ASSESSMENT

ON EXAMINATION

Multiple, superficial engorged veins
May be tender on palpation
Rarely, pelvic examination may reveal tumour causing venous pressure

↓

VARICOSE VEINS

Drain into the deep venous system via connecting or perforating veins in which there are valves
Incompetence of these valves allows transmission, on standing,
of the high pressure in the deep veins to the superficial veins – which then dilate

The main connections are at the sapheno–femoral junction, at perforator veins in the calf
and by the short saphenous vein – at the sapheno–popliteal junction

Establish level of valvular incompetence

Varicosities in short saphenous vein
(passes from popliteal fossa to behind lateral malleolus)

Elevate leg and empty veins
Varicosities DO NOT refill when leg is dependent and
pressure occludes sapheno–popliteal junction

SAPHENO–POPLITEAL JUNCTION INCOMPETENCE

Sapheno–popliteal junction incompetence excluded

TRENDELENBURG TEST:

The leg is elevated, emptying the veins

A tourniquet is applied to the 'emptied' leg and the patient stands
Rapid filling of veins distal to the tourniquet implies
incompetence below that level
The test is repeated at sequential levels
to define the level of valvular incompetence

SAPHENO–FEMORAL JUNCTION INCOMPETENCE

PERFORATOR INCOMPETENCE ONLY

Conservative treatment is advocated, including weight loss and wearing graduated support stockings
Injection sclerotherapy is an option for perforator incompetence

Indications for surgery include cosmesis, pain or discomfort, thrombophlebitis
and (rarely) haemorrhage and ulceration

SURGERY

High tie and ligation of tributaries
Stripping of long saphenous vein

SURGERY

Multiple avulsion of varicosities

SECTION B

UROLOGY

INTRODUCTION

The principal presenting symptoms with which an undergraduate should be familiar are bladder outflow obstruction, retention of urine, bladder instability and haematuria. Acute testicular pain is also an important presenting symptom because many patients are at risk of testicular infarction and the diagnosis is critical. Renal colic, which heralds many 'urological' conditions, is dealt with in Chapter 1.

A typical work-up of a patient presenting with haematuria is illustrated by the following case history.

Case history

A 50-year-old man confides in his daughter, who has recently qualified in medicine, that he is worried about having been passing blood in his urine for 2 weeks. She refers him to a urologist, who further notes that he is overweight and a heavy smoker of long standing and that he has passed clots of blood associated with transient perineal pain. There is no relevant past, family or treatment history and nothing abnormal is found on examination.

1. What does the urologist arrange by way of initial investigation?

On initial investigation it is noted that the urine tests positive for blood and protein. Microscopy and culture reveal red blood cells and a sterile pyuria only, and the sample sent for cytology is reported to be normal.

2. What is the next important investigation?

An intravenous urogram is arranged and the series of films reveals a non-calcified filling defect in the left renal pelvis. The left ureter fills more slowly than the right.

3. What is the most likely diagnosis? What further investigation needs to be done and why?

The urologist suspects a transitional cell tumour of the left kidney and 'clot colic'. He next arranges a retrograde ureterogram to obtain tissue brushings to confirm the diagnosis and at the same time a cystoscopy to exclude coincident bladder tumour.

The histology shows a poorly differentiated transitional cell carcinoma of the renal pelvis, and cystoscopy excludes a bladder tumour.

4. How should this patient be further managed?

17. HAEMATURIA

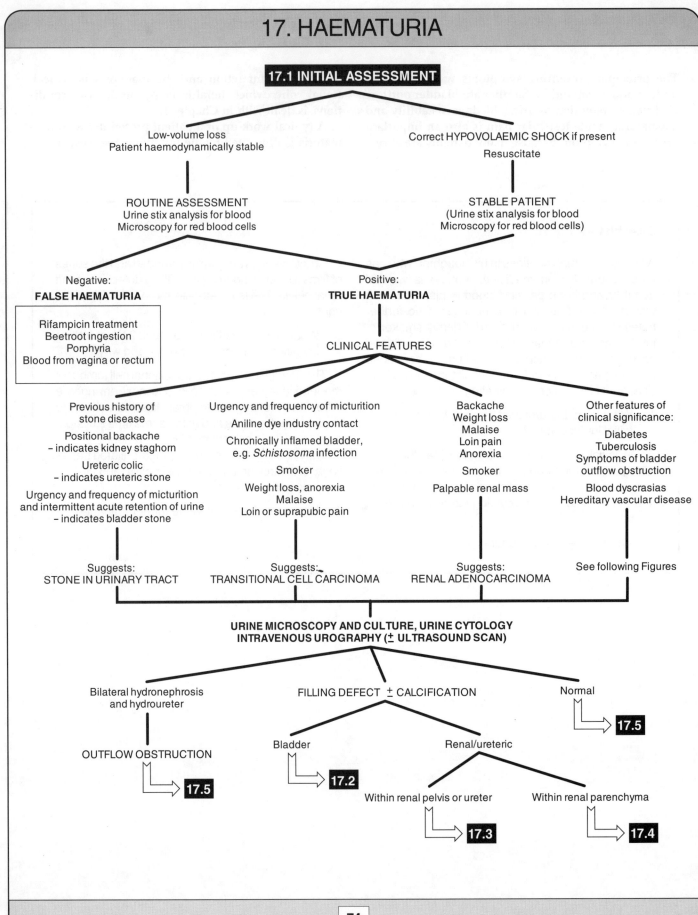

17.1 INITIAL ASSESSMENT

Low-volume loss
Patient haemodynamically stable

Correct HYPOVOLAEMIC SHOCK if present
Resuscitate

ROUTINE ASSESSMENT
Urine stix analysis for blood
Microscopy for red blood cells

STABLE PATIENT
(Urine stix analysis for blood
Microscopy for red blood cells)

Negative:
FALSE HAEMATURIA

Positive:
TRUE HAEMATURIA

Rifampicin treatment
Beetroot ingestion
Porphyria
Blood from vagina or rectum

CLINICAL FEATURES

Previous history of
stone disease

Positional backache
– indicates kidney staghorn

Ureteric colic
– indicates ureteric stone

Urgency and frequency of micturition
and intermittent acute retention of urine
– indicates bladder stone

Suggests:
STONE IN URINARY TRACT

Urgency and frequency of micturition

Aniline dye industry contact

Chronically inflamed bladder,
e.g. *Schistosoma* infection

Smoker

Weight loss, anorexia
Malaise
Loin or suprapubic pain

Suggests:
TRANSITIONAL CELL CARCINOMA

Backache
Weight loss
Malaise
Loin pain
Anorexia

Smoker

Palpable renal mass

Suggests:
RENAL ADENOCARCINOMA

Other features of
clinical significance:

Diabetes
Tuberculosis
Symptoms of bladder
outflow obstruction

Blood dyscrasias
Hereditary vascular disease

See following Figures

URINE MICROSCOPY AND CULTURE, URINE CYTOLOGY
INTRAVENOUS UROGRAPHY ($\pm$ ULTRASOUND SCAN)

Bilateral hydronephrosis
and hydroureter

FILLING DEFECT $\pm$ CALCIFICATION

Normal

OUTFLOW OBSTRUCTION

17.5

Bladder

17.2

Renal/ureteric

17.5

Within renal pelvis or ureter

17.3

Within renal parenchyma

17.4

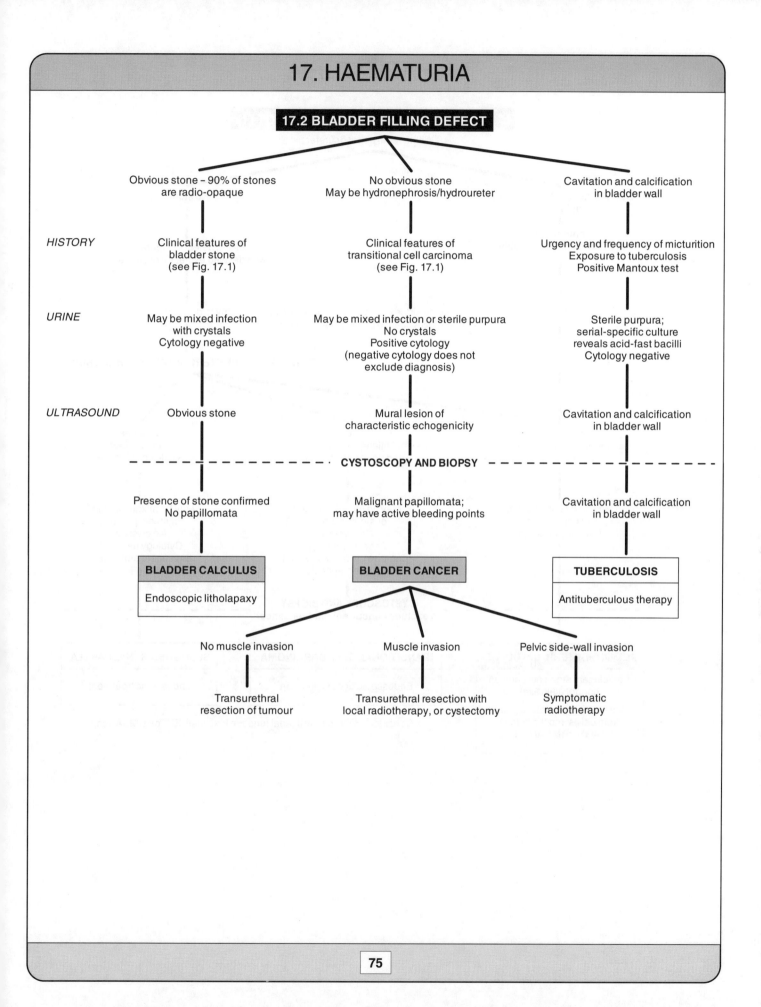

17.2 BLADDER FILLING DEFECT

	Obvious stone – 90% of stones are radio-opaque	No obvious stone May be hydronephrosis/hydroureter	Cavitation and calcification in bladder wall
HISTORY	Clinical features of bladder stone (see Fig. 17.1)	Clinical features of transitional cell carcinoma (see Fig. 17.1)	Urgency and frequency of micturition Exposure to tuberculosis Positive Mantoux test
URINE	May be mixed infection with crystals Cytology negative	May be mixed infection or sterile purpura No crystals Positive cytology (negative cytology does not exclude diagnosis)	Sterile purpura; serial-specific culture reveals acid-fast bacilli Cytology negative
ULTRASOUND	Obvious stone	Mural lesion of characteristic echogenicity	Cavitation and calcification in bladder wall

— — — — — — — — — — **CYSTOSCOPY AND BIOPSY** — — — — — — — — — —

Presence of stone confirmed No papillomata	Malignant papillomata; may have active bleeding points	Cavitation and calcification in bladder wall
BLADDER CALCULUS	**BLADDER CANCER**	**TUBERCULOSIS**
Endoscopic litholapaxy		Antituberculous therapy

No muscle invasion	Muscle invasion	Pelvic side-wall invasion
Transurethral resection of tumour	Transurethral resection with local radiotherapy, or cystectomy	Symptomatic radiotherapy

17. HAEMATURIA

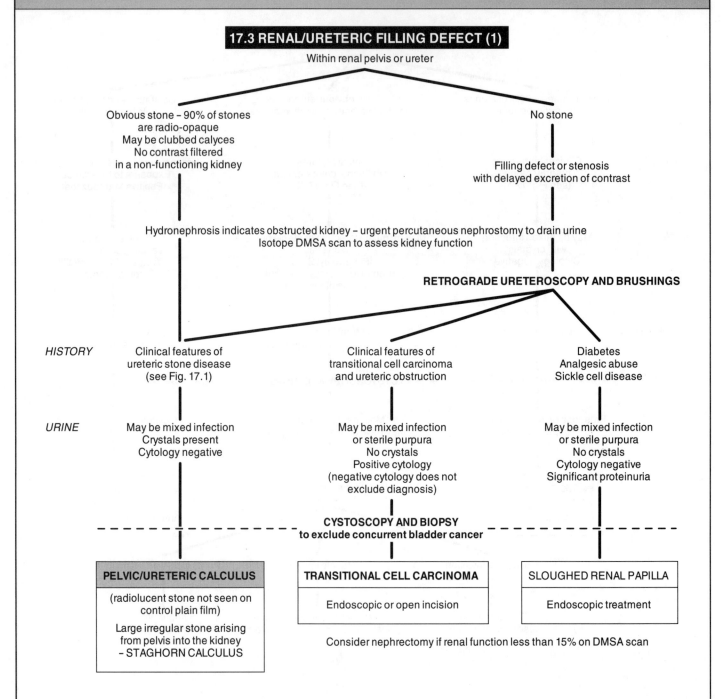

17.3 RENAL/URETERIC FILLING DEFECT (1)

Within renal pelvis or ureter

Obvious stone – 90% of stones
are radio-opaque
May be clubbed calyces
No contrast filtered
in a non-functioning kidney

No stone

Filling defect or stenosis
with delayed excretion of contrast

Hydronephrosis indicates obstructed kidney – urgent percutaneous nephrostomy to drain urine
Isotope DMSA scan to assess kidney function

RETROGRADE URETEROSCOPY AND BRUSHINGS

HISTORY

Clinical features of
ureteric stone disease
(see Fig. 17.1)

Clinical features of
transitional cell carcinoma
and ureteric obstruction

Diabetes
Analgesic abuse
Sickle cell disease

URINE

May be mixed infection
Crystals present
Cytology negative

May be mixed infection
or sterile purpura
No crystals
Positive cytology
(negative cytology does not
exclude diagnosis)

May be mixed infection
or sterile purpura
No crystals
Cytology negative
Significant proteinuria

CYSTOSCOPY AND BIOPSY
to exclude concurrent bladder cancer

PELVIC/URETERIC CALCULUS
(radiolucent stone not seen on control plain film)
Large irregular stone arising from pelvis into the kidney – STAGHORN CALCULUS

TRANSITIONAL CELL CARCINOMA
Endoscopic or open incision

SLOUGHED RENAL PAPILLA
Endoscopic treatment

Consider nephrectomy if renal function less than 15% on DMSA scan

17. HAEMATURIA

17.4 RENAL/URETERIC FILLING DEFECT (2)

Within renal parenchyma

```
Mass lesion distorts            Clubbed calyces            Foci of cavitation and calcification
the pelvicalyceal anatomy       Normal cortex              within normal bladder structure
```

HISTORY

May be clinical features of
renal adenocarcinoma
(see Fig. 17.1)

Diabetes
Analgesic abuse
Sickle cell disease

Exposure to tuberculosis
Positive Mantoux test

URINE

May be mixed infection
Proteinuria
Cytology positive/negative

May be mixed infection or sterile purpura
No crystals
Cytology negative
Significant proteinuria

Sterile purpura;
serial-specific culture
reveals acid-fast bacilli
Cytology negative

CYSTOSCOPY AND BIOPSY
to exclude concurrent bladder cancer

Tumour mass defined by CT scan or
ARTERIOGRAM

| SLOUGHED RENAL PAPILLA |
| Endoscopic treatment |

| **TUBERCULOSIS** |
| Antituberculous therapy |

Perinephric invasion
Tumour circulation

Diagnosis not made

EXCISION BIOPSY

RENAL CELL ADENOCARCINOMA

| **BENIGN TUMOUR, e.g. HAMARTOMA** |
| Nephrectomy |

Tumour within renal capsule

Perinephric and inferior vena cava invasion

Nephrectomy

Nephrectomy for palliation
Radiotherapy for symptomatic metastases

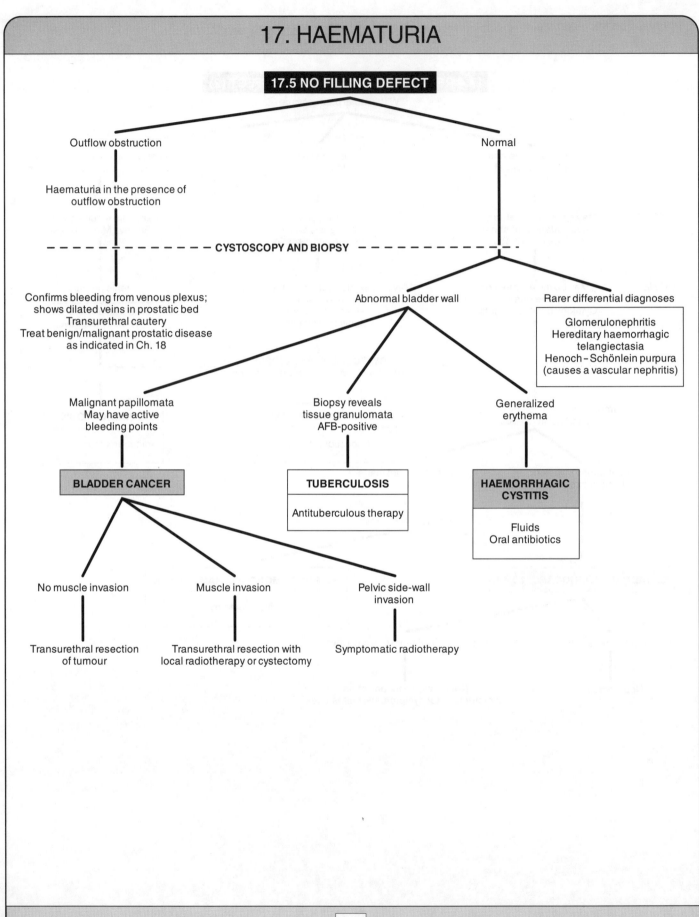

17.5 NO FILLING DEFECT

Outflow obstruction

Haematuria in the presence of outflow obstruction

— — — — — — — — — CYSTOSCOPY AND BIOPSY — — — — — — — —

Confirms bleeding from venous plexus; shows dilated veins in prostatic bed
Transurethral cautery
Treat benign/malignant prostatic disease as indicated in Ch. 18

Normal

Abnormal bladder wall

Rarer differential diagnoses

Glomerulonephritis
Hereditary haemorrhagic telangiectasia
Henoch–Schönlein purpura (causes a vascular nephritis)

Malignant papillomata
May have active bleeding points

BLADDER CANCER

No muscle invasion

Transurethral resection of tumour

Muscle invasion

Transurethral resection with local radiotherapy or cystectomy

Pelvic side-wall invasion

Symptomatic radiotherapy

Biopsy reveals tissue granulomata AFB-positive

TUBERCULOSIS

Antituberculous therapy

Generalized erythema

HAEMORRHAGIC CYSTITIS

Fluids
Oral antibiotics

18. RETENTION OF URINE

18.1 INITIAL ASSESSMENT – MALE PATIENT

PALPABLE BLADDER PER ABDOMEN
Patient has not passed urine
Painful acute retention or chronic painless retention

NEUROLOGICAL ABNORMALITY → **18.4**

No neurological abnormality

If relaxation techniques fail:
URETHRAL CATHETERIZATION

Fails

Successful – symptomatic relief

SUPRAPUBIC CATHETER
Successful – symptomatic relief

CLINICAL FEATURES

Previous symptoms of bladder instability:
– urgency and frequency without
established obstructive symptoms
– burning and stinging on micturition
– haematuria

Suggests:
NON-PROSTATIC
BLADDER OUTFLOW OBSTRUCTION → **18.2**

Previous symptoms of bladder outflow obstruction:
– difficulty in initiating micturition
– urgency and frequency of micturition
– poor stream; postmicturition dribbling
– nocturia; previous acute retention

Usually >50 years old

Suggests:
PROSTATIC OBSTRUCTION

ON EXAMINATION
(rectal examination with empty bladder)

History of constipation
Palpable loaded colon
Faeces per rectum on digital
examination
Abdominal X-ray shows
faecal shadow

CONSTIPATION

Relieve
Remove catheter
Patient passes urine

Normal prostate

Symptoms persist when catheter removed

Large postmicturition residual volume on ULTRASOUND
and LOW FLOW RATE

CYSTOURETHROSCOPY

NON-PROSTATIC BLADDER
OUTFLOW OBSTRUCTION → **18.2**

Large middle lobe of prostate

PROSTATECTOMY
(usually transurethral – TURP)

Large prostate
(may be confirmed by RECTAL ULTRASOUND)

Normal serum acid phosphatase
and prostate-specific antigen
Smooth, soft gland

BENIGN PROSTATIC HYPERTROPHY

Long-standing or recurrent symptoms,
demonstrable postmicturition
residual volume;
proceed to PROSTATECTOMY
(usually transurethral – TURP)

Elevated phosphatase or
specific antigen
Irregular, hard gland

PROSTATIC CANCER

Resect gland
if symptoms persist
Hormone manipulation and
proceed to orchidectomy
if symptomatic metastases

18.2 NON-PROSTATIC BLADDER OUTFLOW OBSTRUCTION

CYSTOURETHROSCOPY/RETROGRADE URETHROGRAPHY

BLADDER NECK OBSTRUCTION

Haematuria
May be clots and 'clot colic'

Clinical features of transitional cell carcinoma

Malignant cells in urine or biopsy tissue

BLADDER CARCINOMA
See p.84

History of:
– sexually transmitted disease
– instrumentation
– perineal trauma
– radiotherapy

BLADDER NECK STRICTURE
Endoscopic release of bladder neck

Clinical feature of bladder stone disease

BLADDER CALCULI
Litholapaxy (stone is crushed by endoscopy and bladder is then irrigated)

URETHRAL OBSTRUCTION

History of:
– sexually transmitted disease
– instrumentation
– perineal trauma
– radiotherapy

Painful ejaculation and micturition

URETHRAL STRICTURE
Urethrotomy

May require several procedures and eventual urethroplasty |

Normal anatomy

Videocystourethrography is diagnostic

Young patient

PRIMARY BLADDER NECK OBSTRUCTION

18. RETENTION OF URINE

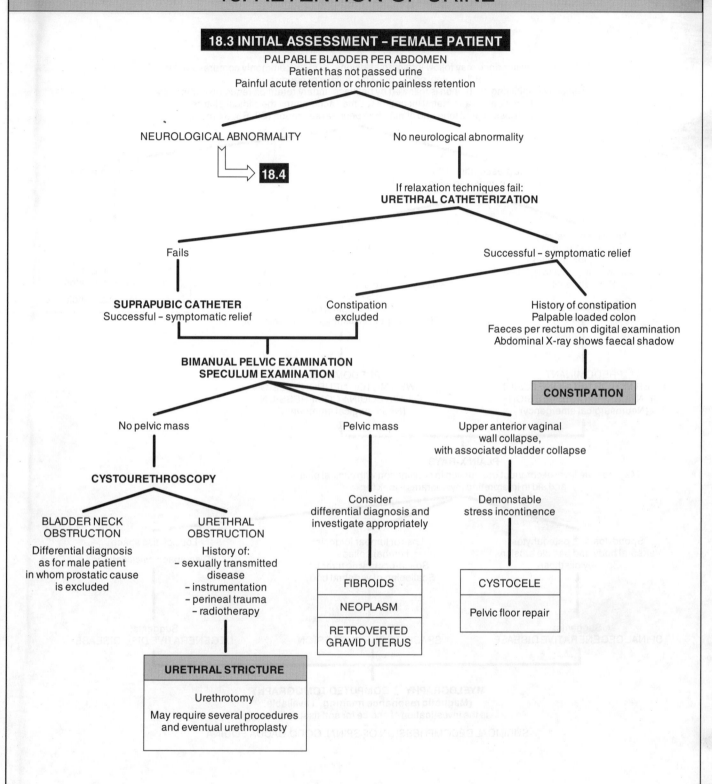

18.3 INITIAL ASSESSMENT – FEMALE PATIENT

PALPABLE BLADDER PER ABDOMEN
Patient has not passed urine
Painful acute retention or chronic painless retention

NEUROLOGICAL ABNORMALITY → **18.4**

No neurological abnormality

If relaxation techniques fail:
URETHRAL CATHETERIZATION

Fails

Successful – symptomatic relief

SUPRAPUBIC CATHETER
Successful – symptomatic relief

Constipation excluded

History of constipation
Palpable loaded colon
Faeces per rectum on digital examination
Abdominal X-ray shows faecal shadow

CONSTIPATION

**BIMANUAL PELVIC EXAMINATION
SPECULUM EXAMINATION**

No pelvic mass

Pelvic mass

Upper anterior vaginal
wall collapse,
with associated bladder collapse

CYSTOURETHROSCOPY

Consider
differential diagnosis and
investigate appropriately

Demonstable
stress incontinence

BLADDER NECK
OBSTRUCTION

Differential diagnosis
as for male patient
in whom prostatic cause
is excluded

URETHRAL
OBSTRUCTION

History of:
– sexually transmitted
disease
– instrumentation
– perineal trauma
– radiotherapy

| FIBROIDS |
| NEOPLASM |
| RETROVERTED GRAVID UTERUS |

| CYSTOCELE |
| Pelvic floor repair |

URETHRAL STRICTURE

Urethrotomy
May require several procedures
and eventual urethroplasty

18. RETENTION OF URINE

18.4 NEUROLOGICAL DISORDER

Sphincter disturbance may follow intracranial lesions, or more commonly compressive lesions
of the spinal cord, conus medullaris or cauda equina
Difficulty in initiating micturition is followed by painless urinary retention requiring catheterization
Constipation and faecal incontinence may accompany the clinical picture,
with loss of anal tone and diminished perineal sensation (S2, S3, S4 roots)

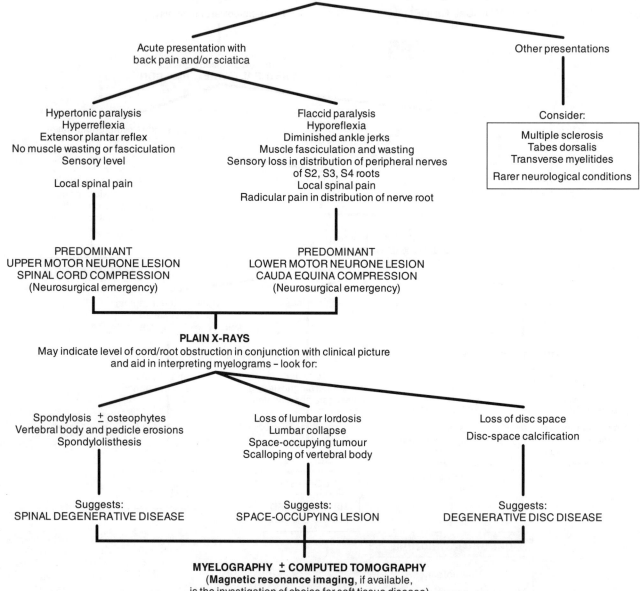

Acute presentation with
back pain and/or sciatica

Other presentations

Hypertonic paralysis
Hyperreflexia
Extensor plantar reflex
No muscle wasting or fasciculation
Sensory level

Local spinal pain

Flaccid paralysis
Hyporeflexia
Diminished ankle jerks
Muscle fasciculation and wasting
Sensory loss in distribution of peripheral nerves
of S2, S3, S4 roots
Local spinal pain
Radicular pain in distribution of nerve root

Consider:

Multiple sclerosis
Tabes dorsalis
Transverse myelitides

Rarer neurological conditions

PREDOMINANT
UPPER MOTOR NEURONE LESION
SPINAL CORD COMPRESSION
(Neurosurgical emergency)

PREDOMINANT
LOWER MOTOR NEURONE LESION
CAUDA EQUINA COMPRESSION
(Neurosurgical emergency)

PLAIN X-RAYS
May indicate level of cord/root obstruction in conjunction with clinical picture
and aid in interpreting myelograms – look for:

Spondylosis ± osteophytes
Vertebral body and pedicle erosions
Spondylolisthesis

Loss of lumbar lordosis
Lumbar collapse
Space-occupying tumour
Scalloping of vertebral body

Loss of disc space
Disc-space calcification

Suggests:
SPINAL DEGENERATIVE DISEASE

Suggests:
SPACE-OCCUPYING LESION

Suggests:
DEGENERATIVE DISC DISEASE

MYELOGRAPHY ± COMPUTED TOMOGRAPHY
(**Magnetic resonance imaging**, if available,
is the investigation of choice for soft tissue disease)

SURGICAL DECOMPRESSION OF SPINAL CORD/CAUDA EQUINA

19. ACUTE TESTICULAR PAIN

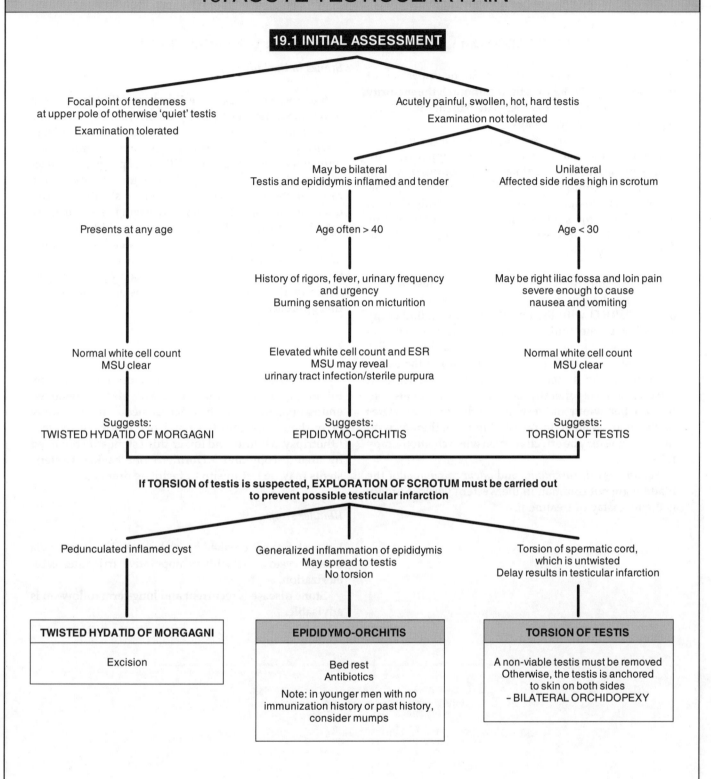

19.1 INITIAL ASSESSMENT

Focal point of tenderness at upper pole of otherwise 'quiet' testis
Examination tolerated

Acutely painful, swollen, hot, hard testis
Examination not tolerated

May be bilateral
Testis and epididymis inflamed and tender

Unilateral
Affected side rides high in scrotum

Presents at any age

Age often > 40

Age < 30

History of rigors, fever, urinary frequency and urgency
Burning sensation on micturition

May be right iliac fossa and loin pain severe enough to cause nausea and vomiting

Normal white cell count
MSU clear

Elevated white cell count and ESR
MSU may reveal urinary tract infection/sterile purpura

Normal white cell count
MSU clear

Suggests:
TWISTED HYDATID OF MORGAGNI

Suggests:
EPIDIDYMO-ORCHITIS

Suggests:
TORSION OF TESTIS

If TORSION of testis is suspected, EXPLORATION OF SCROTUM must be carried out to prevent possible testicular infarction

Pedunculated inflamed cyst

Generalized inflammation of epididymis
May spread to testis
No torsion

Torsion of spermatic cord, which is untwisted
Delay results in testicular infarction

TWISTED HYDATID OF MORGAGNI

Excision

EPIDIDYMO-ORCHITIS

Bed rest
Antibiotics

Note: in younger men with no immunization history or past history, consider mumps

TORSION OF TESTIS

A non-viable testis must be removed
Otherwise, the testis is anchored to skin on both sides
– BILATERAL ORCHIDOPEXY

TRANSITIONAL CELL CARCINOMA

Isolated transitional cell carcinoma in the upper part of the tract is rare (38% of urethral tumours); the majority of cases occur in the bladder. All patients thus have regular follow-up cystoscopy.

Radical nephro-ureterectomy is considered for high-grade, multifocal and muscle-invasive upper tract tumours by open excision, alone or in combination with endoscopic techniques. Conservative surgery (e.g. partial open or endoscopic resection of kidney and/or ureter) is considered for solitary tumours, especially of low grade and stage, and where the renal function is poor. Unnecessarily radical treatment will prejudice options later.

Bladder transitional cell carcinoma is resected by endoscopic transurethral resection of the bladder tumour (TURBT) with the use of adjuvant radiotherapy according to the tumour histology. Further management options for aggressive or multifocal tumours include cystectomy and urinary diversion, and the use of intravesical and systemic chemotherapy. Transitional cell carcinoma is generally more radio- and chemosensitive; the behaviour and response of the tumour dictates further management. Intravesical immunotherapy with BCG vaccine may be effective, even when chemotherapy fails.

Squamous cell carcinoma and *adenocarcinoma* of the bladder are not common in the western world. Surgery is the mainstay of treatment.

CALCULI IN THE RENAL TRACT

Stones in the kidney

Extracorporeal shock-wave lithotripsy (ESWL) is used to fragment the stones, using pulsing shock waves in a water bath or under ultrasound guidance with piezo-electric generated pulses. ESWL is used in combination with percutaneous surgery. Dilators of progressive magnitude are passed over a guide wire into the lower pole calyx of the prone patient. A plastic sheath is introduced and the stones are removed leaving a nephrostomy tube in situ for 24–48 hours to drain the kidney.

Endoscopic renal surgery techniques allow treatment of 90% of stones. Occasionally, however, caliceal stag-horn calculi may be removed by open operation, particularly if there are other circumstances favouring this approach.

Ureteric stones

Upper and lower third stones may be fragmented by lithotripsy. Upper third stones may also be removed endoscopically through a percutaneous nephrostomy or pushed back into the renal pelvis for subsequent lithotripsy. Middle- and lower-third stones are removed by ureteroscopy and a Dornier stone basket. Ureteric stents may be left in situ to facilitate drainage.

Bladder stones

Large stones are crushed by endoscopic litholapaxy via a rigid cystoscope with postoperative irrigating catheterization.

Stone disease is recurrent and long-term follow-up is advisable.

SECTION C

ORTHOPAEDICS AND TRAUMA

20. PRINCIPLES OF FRACTURE MANAGEMENT

INTRODUCTION

A fracture is a break in the continuity of a bone. The clinical features are:

a. pain and tenderness
b. local swelling and bruising
c. crepitus over the site of pain
d. deformity and abnormal mobility
e. loss of normal function

Fractures have three causes:

a. *traumatic fractures* – normal bone, abnormal forces
b. *fatigue* or *stress fractures* – repetitive insult
c. *pathological fractures* – abnormal bone, normal forces

Healing of a fracture happens in the following sequence:

1. haematoma formation
2. organization of the haematoma
3. callus formation (of woven bone) – visible on X-ray
4. consolidation by mature bone (lamellar bone)
5. remodelling

When consolidation occurs a fracture is said to be secure.

Time for fracture healing:

a. cancellous bone takes approximately 6 weeks to heal
b. cortical bone takes approximately 12 weeks to heal
c. children's fractures generally take half the time of adult fractures to heal
d. upper limb fractures take half the time of lower limb fractures to heal

20. PRINCIPLES OF FRACTURE MANAGEMENT

20.1 INITIAL ASSESSMENT

CORRECT HYPOVOLAEMIC SHOCK (see Ch. 22)

Skin breached

COMPOUND FRACTURE
Tetanus prophylaxis
Antibiotics

Absent pulse distal to fracture
Altered neurology distal to fracture

Neurovascular damage

Urgent exploration in theatre
→ **20.4**

Skin not breached

CLOSED FRACTURE
X-ray in more than one plane;
this may be compared to uninjured side

No neurovascular damage
X-ray shows:

More than two fragments
– COMMINUTED FRACTURE

Two fragments only
– NOT COMMINUTED FRACTURE

Bones not aligned
– DISPLACED FRACTURE

Bones correctly aligned
– UNDISPLACED FRACTURE
Immobilize until union has occurred,
e.g. PLASTER FIXATION

Fragments not in line
but parallel
– MALAPPOSITION

Rotation of distal fragment
on proximal one
– MALROTATION

Fragments not parallel and ends meet,
creating an angle
– MALALIGNMENT

Fragments parallel
but overlapping
– DISPLACEMENT OF LENGTH
(SHORTENING)

Any one or combination of the above
REDUCTION REQUIRED

Intra-articular fracture
Multiple trauma
Pathological fractures
Fractures prone to non-union, e.g. femoral neck
Fractures prone to malunion,
e.g. fracture subluxations of the ankle and wrist
or mid-shaft fractures of the forearm

Non-articular fractures
Simple trauma

OPEN REDUCTION usually required
→ **20.3**

CLOSED REDUCTION may be attempted
→ **20.2**

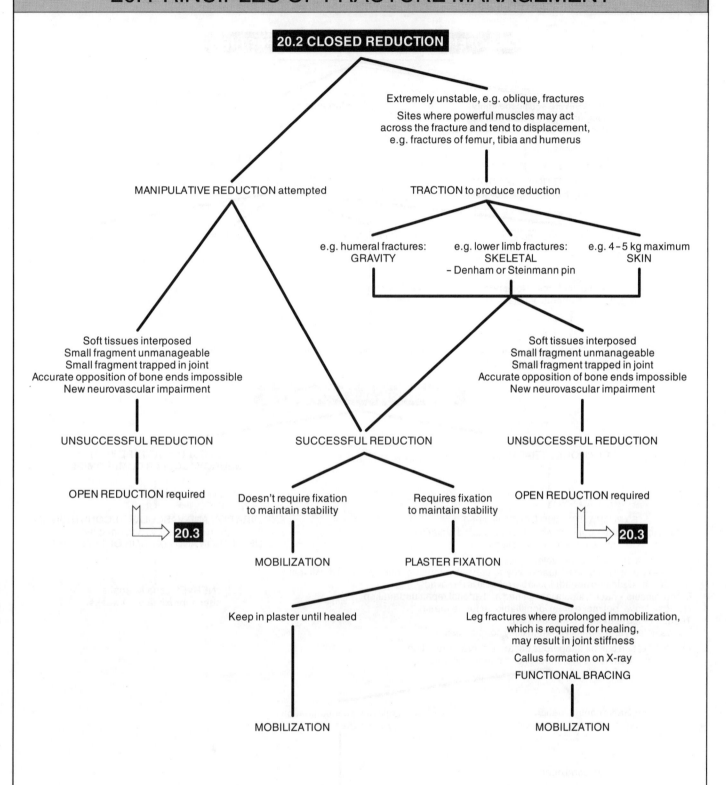

20.2 CLOSED REDUCTION

Extremely unstable, e.g. oblique, fractures

Sites where powerful muscles may act
across the fracture and tend to displacement,
e.g. fractures of femur, tibia and humerus

MANIPULATIVE REDUCTION attempted

TRACTION to produce reduction

e.g. humeral fractures:
GRAVITY

e.g. lower limb fractures:
SKELETAL
– Denham or Steinmann pin

e.g. 4–5 kg maximum
SKIN

Soft tissues interposed
Small fragment unmanageable
Small fragment trapped in joint
Accurate opposition of bone ends impossible
New neurovascular impairment

Soft tissues interposed
Small fragment unmanageable
Small fragment trapped in joint
Accurate opposition of bone ends impossible
New neurovascular impairment

UNSUCCESSFUL REDUCTION

SUCCESSFUL REDUCTION

UNSUCCESSFUL REDUCTION

OPEN REDUCTION required

20.3

Doesn't require fixation
to maintain stability

Requires fixation
to maintain stability

OPEN REDUCTION required

20.3

MOBILIZATION

PLASTER FIXATION

Keep in plaster until healed

Leg fractures where prolonged immobilization,
which is required for healing,
may result in joint stiffness

Callus formation on X-ray

FUNCTIONAL BRACING

MOBILIZATION

MOBILIZATION

20. PRINCIPLES OF FRACTURE MANAGEMENT

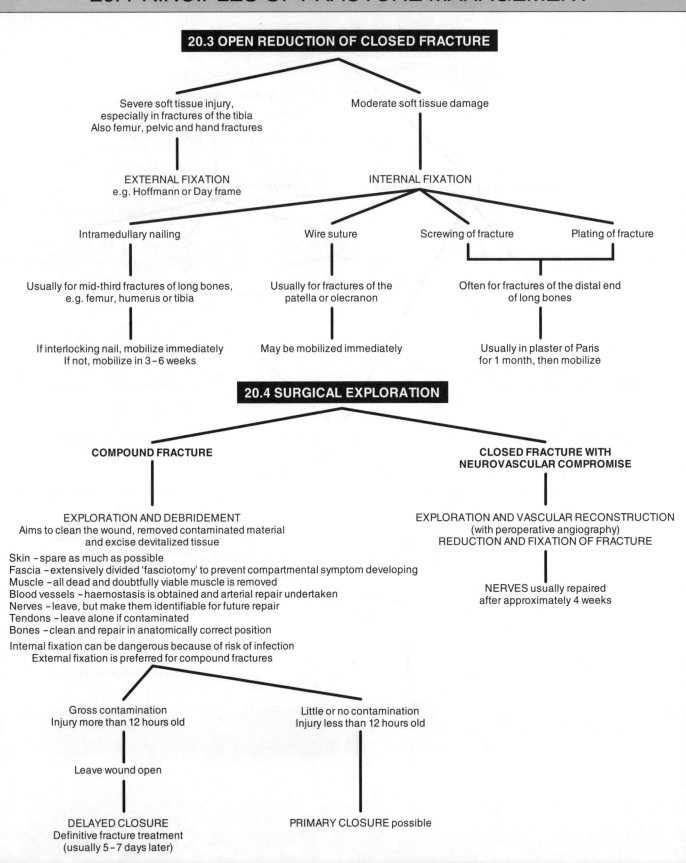

20.3 OPEN REDUCTION OF CLOSED FRACTURE

Severe soft tissue injury, especially in fractures of the tibia
Also femur, pelvic and hand fractures

Moderate soft tissue damage

EXTERNAL FIXATION
e.g. Hoffmann or Day frame

INTERNAL FIXATION

Intramedullary nailing

Wire suture

Screwing of fracture

Plating of fracture

Usually for mid-third fractures of long bones, e.g. femur, humerus or tibia

Usually for fractures of the patella or olecranon

Often for fractures of the distal end of long bones

If interlocking nail, mobilize immediately
If not, mobilize in 3–6 weeks

May be mobilized immediately

Usually in plaster of Paris for 1 month, then mobilize

20.4 SURGICAL EXPLORATION

COMPOUND FRACTURE

CLOSED FRACTURE WITH NEUROVASCULAR COMPROMISE

EXPLORATION AND DEBRIDEMENT
Aims to clean the wound, removed contaminated material and excise devitalized tissue

Skin – spare as much as possible
Fascia – extensively divided 'fasciotomy' to prevent compartmental symptom developing
Muscle – all dead and doubtfully viable muscle is removed
Blood vessels – haemostasis is obtained and arterial repair undertaken
Nerves – leave, but make them identifiable for future repair
Tendons – leave alone if contaminated
Bones – clean and repair in anatomically correct position

Internal fixation can be dangerous because of risk of infection
External fixation is preferred for compound fractures

EXPLORATION AND VASCULAR RECONSTRUCTION
(with peroperative angiography)
REDUCTION AND FIXATION OF FRACTURE

NERVES usually repaired
after approximately 4 weeks

Gross contamination
Injury more than 12 hours old

Little or no contamination
Injury less than 12 hours old

Leave wound open

DELAYED CLOSURE
Definitive fracture treatment
(usually 5–7 days later)

PRIMARY CLOSURE possible

INTRODUCTION

Head injuries are relevant because of the brain injuries following them. These are either primary (occurring at the time of impact) or secondary (resulting from a chain of events triggered by the initial injury). The cranial vault acts as a closed box, within which blood or swelling soon results in raised intracranial pressure and compression of healthy brain.

The most important aspect of the management of head injuries is the prevention, or early recognition and treatment, of secondary brain injury.

Signs of raised intracranial pressure are:

a. falling pulse rate
b. rising blood pressure
c. slowing and reduced depth of breathing
d. decreasing Glasgow coma score
e. dilatation, loss of light reaction or asymmetry of pupils

The clinical signs of skull fracture are:

a. periorbital haematoma (panda eye)
b. bruising over the mastoid area (Battle's sign)
c. cerebrospinal fluid leaking from the nose, the ear and lacerations overlying fractures
d. boggy scalp swellings
e. subconjunctival haemorrhage with no posterior limit

Case history

A 24-year-old lady who has been in a road traffic accident arrives at your Accident and Emergency Department with an isolated head injury.

On examination she opens her eyes when you address her. She can tell you her name and address and localizes painful stimuli.

1. What is her Glasgow coma score?

Her pupils are equal and react to light. She has equal power on right and left. There are no lacerations or depressions in the skull and scalp but there is fluid running from her nose. She also has bilateral periorbital haematomas.

2. What is the relevance of the fluid running from her nose?

3. How would you investigate if cerebrospinal fluid is present in this fluid?

4. On opening her eyes, what sign is likely to be present?

The patient is admitted to hospital.

5. Would you perform a CT scan in this case?

CT shows no intracerebral haematoma which requires drainage but confirms the presence of an anterior fossa fracture.

6. Does this patient warrant antibiotics?

7. Why is it dangerous to try to pass a nasogastric tube in this case?

8. What material may be used to close the dural tear if it does not close spontaneously?

21. HEAD INJURY

21.1 INITIAL ASSESSMENT

ENSURE PRIMARY SURVEY IS COMPLETED
(see Ch. 22)

ASSESS LEVEL OF CONSCIOUSNESS using Glasgow Coma Scale

Eye opening response:	Spontaneously – already open with blinking	4
	To speech	3
	To stimulus	2
	None	1
Best motor response:	Obeys – moves limbs to command	6
	Purposeful movement – moves towards painful stimulus	5
	Withdraws – pulls away from painful stimulus	4
	Abnormal flexion – decorticate posture	3
	Extensor response – decerebrate posture	2
	No movement	1
Verbal response:	Orientated	5
	Confused conversation – still answers questions	4
	Inappropriate words – speech random	3
	Incomprehensible sounds – grunts and groans	2
	None	1

TOTAL SCORE

Glasgow Coma Scale ≤8

Glasgow Coma Scale >8 → 21.2

Pupils equal
No asymmetrical abnormal neurology

Pupils unequal
Asymmetrical abnormal neurology

Suspect:
DIFFUSE AXONAL INJURY

Suspect:
INTRACRANIAL BLEED

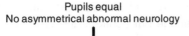

Immediate CT SCAN

No intracranial
space-occupying lesion

INTRACRANIAL BLEED

PRIMARY BRAIN INJURY

Admit
Intubate and ventilate if unable to
support own oxygenation
Mannitol
If CT signs of raised
intracranial pressure,
insert intracranial pressure bolt

ACUTE EXTRADURAL HAEMATOMA | ACUTE SUBDURAL HAEMATOMA

Admit
Intubate and hyperventilate
to optimize cerebral oxygenation
Mannitol
Urgent evacuation

ACUTE INTRACEREBRAL BLEED

Admit
Intubate and hyperventilate
to optimize cerebral oxygenation
If CT signs of raised
intracranial pressure,
consider urgent evacuation;
if not, intracranial bolt to
monitor intracranial pressure

21. HEAD INJURY

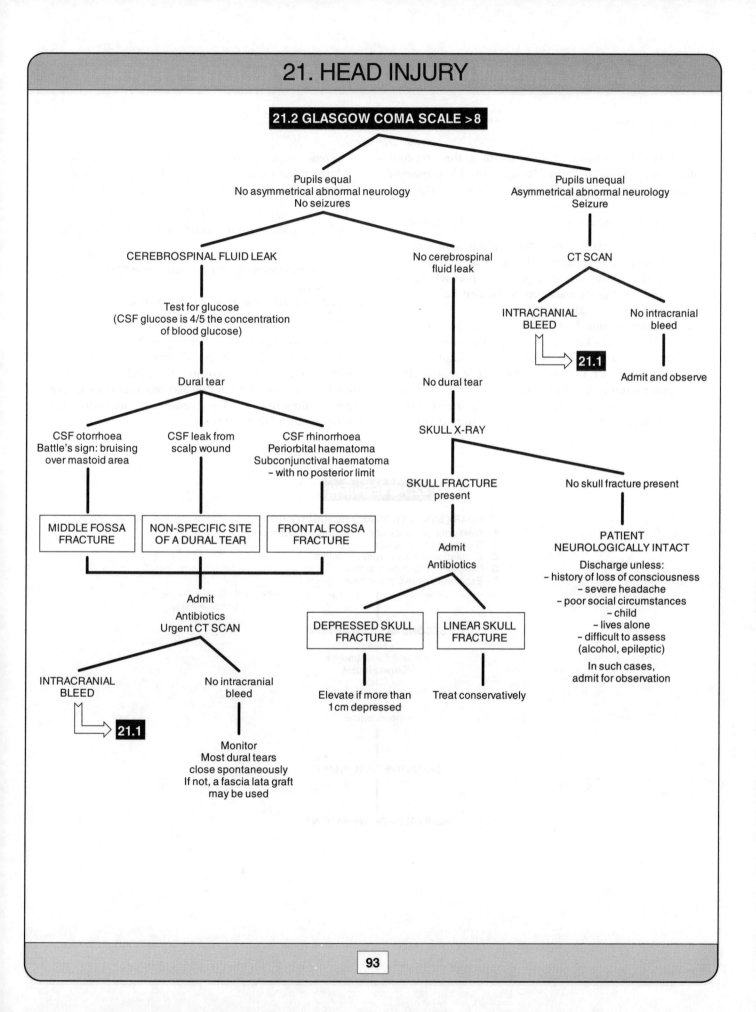

21.2 GLASGOW COMA SCALE >8

Pupils equal
No asymmetrical abnormal neurology
No seizures

Pupils unequal
Asymmetrical abnormal neurology
Seizure

CEREBROSPINAL FLUID LEAK

No cerebrospinal fluid leak

CT SCAN

INTRACRANIAL BLEED → 21.1

No intracranial bleed

Admit and observe

Test for glucose
(CSF glucose is 4/5 the concentration of blood glucose)

Dural tear

No dural tear

SKULL X-RAY

CSF otorrhoea
Battle's sign: bruising over mastoid area

CSF leak from scalp wound

CSF rhinorrhoea
Periorbital haematoma
Subconjunctival haematoma
– with no posterior limit

SKULL FRACTURE present

No skull fracture present

MIDDLE FOSSA FRACTURE

NON-SPECIFIC SITE OF A DURAL TEAR

FRONTAL FOSSA FRACTURE

Admit
Antibiotics

PATIENT NEUROLOGICALLY INTACT

Discharge unless:
– history of loss of consciousness
– severe headache
– poor social circumstances
– child
– lives alone
– difficult to assess (alcohol, epileptic)

In such cases, admit for observation

Admit
Antibiotics
Urgent CT SCAN

DEPRESSED SKULL FRACTURE

LINEAR SKULL FRACTURE

INTRACRANIAL BLEED → 21.1

No intracranial bleed

Elevate if more than 1 cm depressed

Treat conservatively

Monitor
Most dural tears close spontaneously
If not, a fascia lata graft may be used

93

INTRODUCTION

Trauma is the leading cause of death in the first four decades of life in the United Kingdom and is surpassed only by cancer and atherosclerosis as a cause of death in the elderly.

Death from injury follows a trimodal distribution:

1. *Injuries causing death within seconds to minutes*: Most of these patients will die; those that are saved include patients injured in areas where rapid emergency transport and expert help are immediately available.
2. *Injuries causing death within minutes to hours*: This period is known as the 'golden hour': many of these patients can be saved. This chapter deals primarily with the injuries that cause morbidity and mortality in this period.
3. *Injuries causing death days to weeks later*: the two commonest causes of death in this period are sepsis and organ failure. The incidence of these late problems may be reduced by effective and correct initial treatment in the golden hour.

Effective management of the multiple-injured patient in the golden hour should be structured around:

1. *primary survey and resuscitation* – the identification and treatment of immediate life-threatening injuries
2. *secondary survey* in which other injuries are documented and attended to

Peritoneal lavage is a technique that enables the clinician to investigate the possibility of intraperitoneal bleeding. Warm normal saline is instilled into the peritoneal cavity. More than 100 000 red blood cells per cubic millimetre of the fluid removed is an indication for exploratory laparotomy.

22.1 OVERVIEW

PRIMARY EVALUATION AND RESUSCITATION
A – Airway maintenance with cervical spine protection
B – Breathing and ventilation
C – Circulation with haemorrhage control
D – Disability: neurological status
E – Exposure: remove all clothing

|

SECONDARY EVALUATION
– Head
– Maxillofacial trauma
– Cervical spine
– Chest
– Abdomen
– Fractures
– Neurological

|

DEFINITIVE CARE PHASE

|

RE-EVALUATE THE PATIENT

Case history

A 21-year-old man arrives in the Accident and Emergency Department. The ambulance crew say he was involved in a road traffic accident 35 minutes ago. He is unconscious. On examination he is cyanosed and has a respiratory rate of 33, a heart rate of 134 and a blood pressure of 85/40. He has no obvious facial injuries.

1. Should this patient have a cervical collar on?

2. Would you intubate him?

   The findings on examination of his chest are:
   a. there is no open chest wound
   b. the trachea is displaced to the left
   c. there are distended neck veins on the left
   d. the percussion note is hyperresonant on the left and dull on the right
   e. there is decreased air entry on both sides

3. What is the likely diagnosis to account for the left-sided signs?

4. What initial treatment should be initiated?

5. What further treatment is necessary?

6. What is the likely diagnosis to account for the right-sided signs?

7. What treatment is indicated?

8. Where would you insert these intercostal drains?

9. 270 ml of blood is drained from the right side. Is this an indication for a formal thoracotomy?

   The patient's respiratory distress is now decreasing. He has one large intravenous line in his left antecubital fossa.

10. Would you put up another line?

11. How much and what fluid would you give intravenously?

    The patient's blood pressure increases, with a maximum systolic of 110 mmHg, followed by a slow, steady decline.

12. What fluid would you use to replace this continuing loss?

    The patient responds to painful stimuli; the pupils are equal and react briskly to light.

13. What X-rays would you order now?

    These are taken and a nasogastric tube is passed. You decide to pass a urinary catheter.

14. What four examination findings would you note before passing the catheter?

    The secondary survey is started. The patient's Glasgow coma score is 13.
    The respiratory function remains stable and there is no further drainage of blood from the right intercostal drain. The blood pressure and pulse remain unstable (i.e. if the intravenous infusion is slowed down the blood pressure falls and the pulse rate increases). The chest X-ray is normal. Abdominal examination is unrewarding.

15. Would you perform a diagnostic peritoneal lavage on this patient?

    The diagnostic lavage is positive.

16. Should this patient be taken directly to theatre or not?

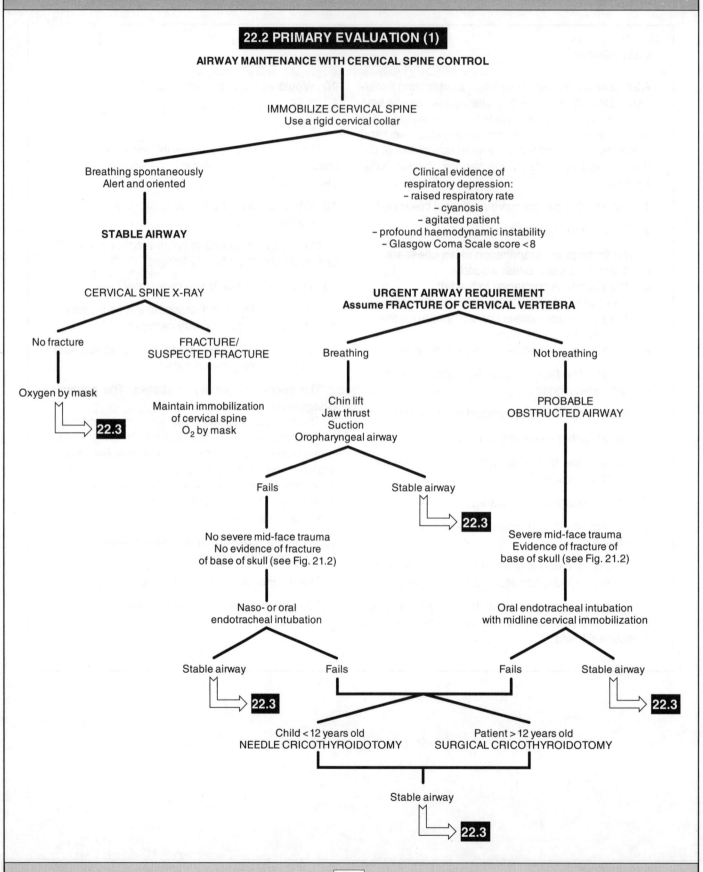

22.2 PRIMARY EVALUATION (1)

AIRWAY MAINTENANCE WITH CERVICAL SPINE CONTROL

IMMOBILIZE CERVICAL SPINE
Use a rigid cervical collar

Breathing spontaneously
Alert and oriented

STABLE AIRWAY

CERVICAL SPINE X-RAY

No fracture

FRACTURE/
SUSPECTED FRACTURE

Oxygen by mask

→ 22.3

Maintain immobilization
of cervical spine
O_2 by mask

Clinical evidence of
respiratory depression:
– raised respiratory rate
– cyanosis
– agitated patient
– profound haemodynamic instability
– Glasgow Coma Scale score <8

URGENT AIRWAY REQUIREMENT
Assume FRACTURE OF CERVICAL VERTEBRA

Breathing

Not breathing

Chin lift
Jaw thrust
Suction
Oropharyngeal airway

PROBABLE
OBSTRUCTED AIRWAY

Fails

Stable airway

→ 22.3

No severe mid-face trauma
No evidence of fracture
of base of skull (see Fig. 21.2)

Severe mid-face trauma
Evidence of fracture of
base of skull (see Fig. 21.2)

Naso- or oral
endotracheal intubation

Oral endotracheal intubation
with midline cervical immobilization

Stable airway

Fails

Fails

Stable airway

→ 22.3

→ 22.3

Child < 12 years old
NEEDLE CRICOTHYROIDOTOMY

Patient > 12 years old
SURGICAL CRICOTHYROIDOTOMY

Stable airway

→ 22.3

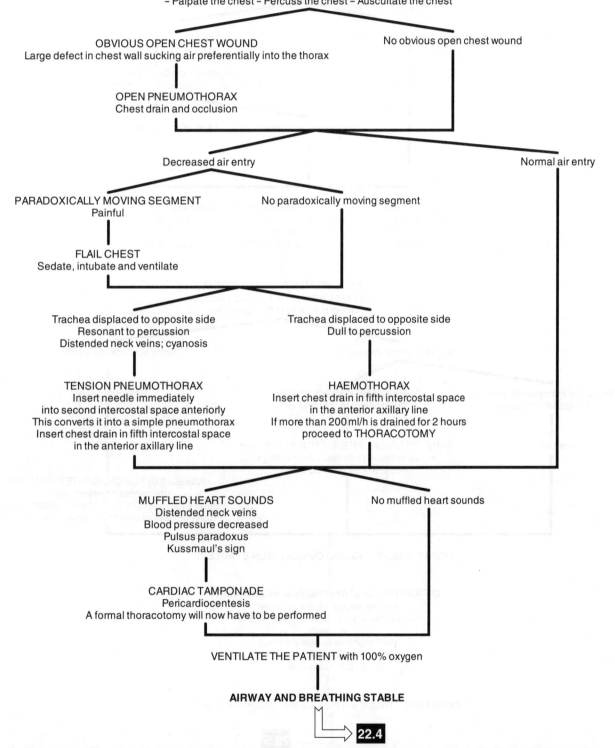

22.3 PRIMARY EVALUATION (2)

BREATHING AND VENTILATION
Expose the whole chest
Examination: Inspect the chest and neck veins
– Assess rate and depth of ventilation – Check position of trachea
– Palpate the chest – Percuss the chest – Auscultate the chest

OBVIOUS OPEN CHEST WOUND
Large defect in chest wall sucking air preferentially into the thorax

No obvious open chest wound

OPEN PNEUMOTHORAX
Chest drain and occlusion

Decreased air entry

Normal air entry

PARADOXICALLY MOVING SEGMENT
Painful

No paradoxically moving segment

FLAIL CHEST
Sedate, intubate and ventilate

Trachea displaced to opposite side
Resonant to percussion
Distended neck veins; cyanosis

Trachea displaced to opposite side
Dull to percussion

TENSION PNEUMOTHORAX
Insert needle immediately
into second intercostal space anteriorly
This converts it into a simple pneumothorax
Insert chest drain in fifth intercostal space
in the anterior axillary line

HAEMOTHORAX
Insert chest drain in fifth intercostal space
in the anterior axillary line
If more than 200 ml/h is drained for 2 hours
proceed to THORACOTOMY

MUFFLED HEART SOUNDS
Distended neck veins
Blood pressure decreased
Pulsus paradoxus
Kussmaul's sign

No muffled heart sounds

CARDIAC TAMPONADE
Pericardiocentesis
A formal thoracotomy will now have to be performed

VENTILATE THE PATIENT with 100% oxygen

AIRWAY AND BREATHING STABLE

→ 22.4

22.4 PRIMARY EVALUATION (3)

CIRCULATION AND HAEMORRHAGE CONTROL
Insert two large intravenous catheters
Assess: Blood loss – Pulse rate – Blood pressure – Pulse pressure – Respiratory rate – Urine output
Take FBC, U & E, cross-match, glucose, amylase

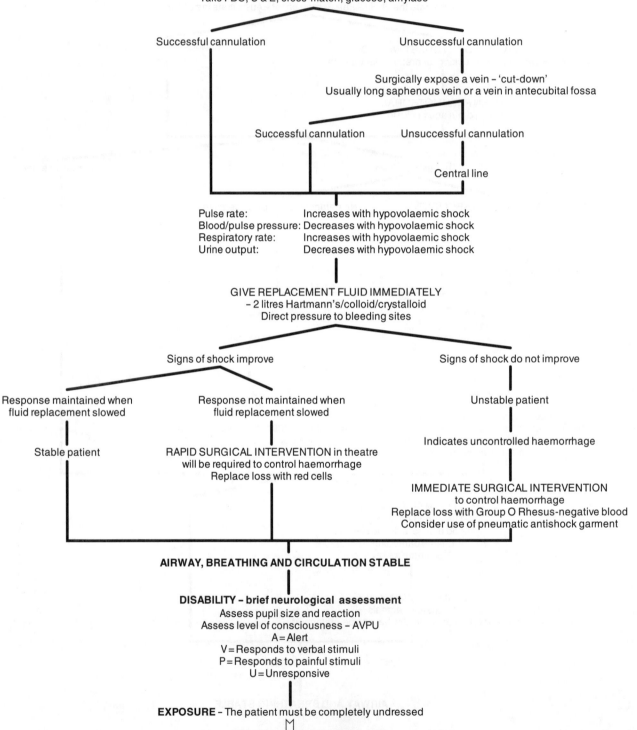

Successful cannulation

Unsuccessful cannulation

Surgically expose a vein – 'cut-down'
Usually long saphenous vein or a vein in antecubital fossa

Successful cannulation   Unsussessful cannulation

Central line

Pulse rate: Increases with hypovolaemic shock
Blood/pulse pressure: Decreases with hypovolaemic shock
Respiratory rate: Increases with hypovolaemic shock
Urine output: Decreases with hypovolaemic shock

GIVE REPLACEMENT FLUID IMMEDIATELY
– 2 litres Hartmann's/colloid/crystalloid
Direct pressure to bleeding sites

Signs of shock improve   Signs of shock do not improve

Response maintained when   Response not maintained when   Unstable patient
fluid replacement slowed   fluid replacement slowed

Stable patient   RAPID SURGICAL INTERVENTION in theatre   Indicates uncontrolled haemorrhage
                   will be required to control haemorrhage
                   Replace loss with red cells

                                                IMMEDIATE SURGICAL INTERVENTION
                                                to control haemorrhage
                                                Replace loss with Group O Rhesus-negative blood
                                                Consider use of pneumatic antishock garment

AIRWAY, BREATHING AND CIRCULATION STABLE

DISABILITY – brief neurological assessment
Assess pupil size and reaction
Assess level of consciousness – AVPU
A = Alert
V = Responds to verbal stimuli
P = Responds to painful stimuli
U = Unresponsive

EXPOSURE – The patient must be completely undressed

22.5

22.5 PRIMARY SURVEY AND IMMEDIATE RESUSCITATION COMPLETE

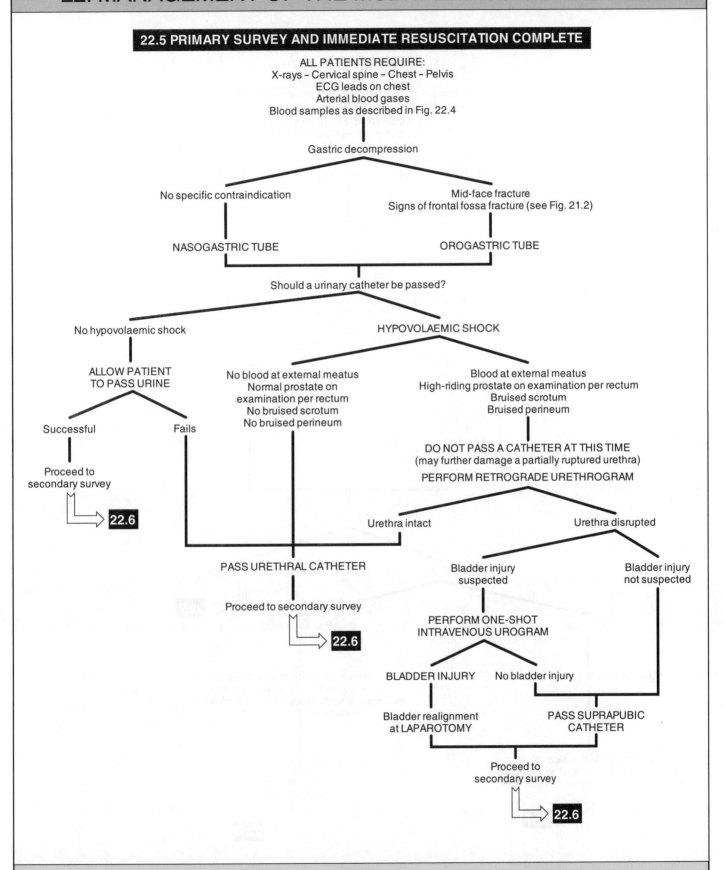

ALL PATIENTS REQUIRE:
X-rays – Cervical spine – Chest – Pelvis
ECG leads on chest
Arterial blood gases
Blood samples as described in Fig. 22.4

Gastric decompression

No specific contraindication

Mid-face fracture
Signs of frontal fossa fracture (see Fig. 21.2)

NASOGASTRIC TUBE

OROGASTRIC TUBE

Should a urinary catheter be passed?

No hypovolaemic shock

HYPOVOLAEMIC SHOCK

ALLOW PATIENT
TO PASS URINE

No blood at external meatus
Normal prostate on
examination per rectum
No bruised scrotum
No bruised perineum

Blood at external meatus
High-riding prostate on examination per rectum
Bruised scrotum
Bruised perineum

Successful

Fails

DO NOT PASS A CATHETER AT THIS TIME
(may further damage a partially ruptured urethra)
PERFORM RETROGRADE URETHROGRAM

Proceed to
secondary survey

22.6

Urethra intact

Urethra disrupted

PASS URETHRAL CATHETER

Bladder injury
suspected

Bladder injury
not suspected

Proceed to secondary survey

22.6

PERFORM ONE-SHOT
INTRAVENOUS UROGRAM

BLADDER INJURY

No bladder injury

Bladder realignment
at LAPAROTOMY

PASS SUPRAPUBIC
CATHETER

Proceed to
secondary survey

22.6

22.6 SECONDARY EVALUATION (1)

HEAD INJURY (see Ch. 21)

Assess **FACIAL INJURY**
– maxillofacial injuries not associated with airway obstruction
are dealt with when the patient's condition is stable

Check **CERVICAL SPINE STABILITY**
This X-ray must show all the cervical vertebral bodies
and intravertebral disc spaces
including the C7 – T1 junction

If at all unsure that the X-ray is normal, leave the collar on

THORACIC TRAUMA:
A chest X-ray is essential
Repeat the examination of the chest:
– Inspect the chest and neck veins
– Assess rate and depth of ventilation
– Check position of trachea
– Palpate the chest and neck for surgical emphysema
– Percuss the chest
– Auscultate the chest

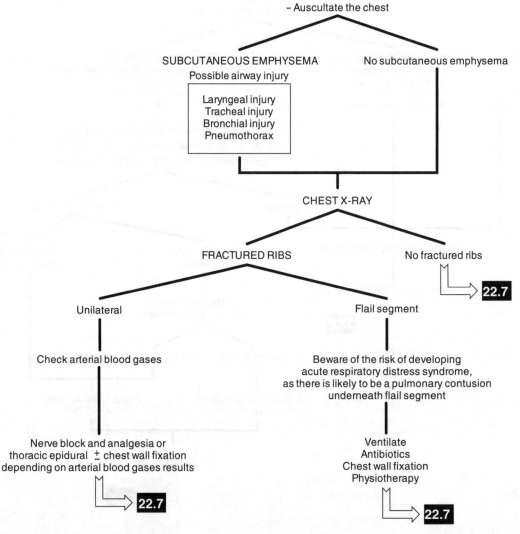

SUBCUTANEOUS EMPHYSEMA
Possible airway injury

Laryngeal injury
Tracheal injury
Bronchial injury
Pneumothorax

No subcutaneous emphysema

CHEST X-RAY

FRACTURED RIBS

No fractured ribs

22.7

Unilateral

Flail segment

Check arterial blood gases

Beware of the risk of developing
acute respiratory distress syndrome,
as there is likely to be a pulmonary contusion
underneath flail segment

Nerve block and analgesia or
thoracic epidural ± chest wall fixation
depending on arterial blood gases results

22.7

Ventilate
Antibiotics
Chest wall fixation
Physiotherapy

22.7

22.7 SECONDARY EVALUATION (2)

PRIMARY SURVEY AND IMMEDIATE RESUSCITATION complete
HEAD INJURY assessed and treated
FACIAL INJURY assessed
CERVICAL INJURY assessed
THORACIC TRAUMA assessed

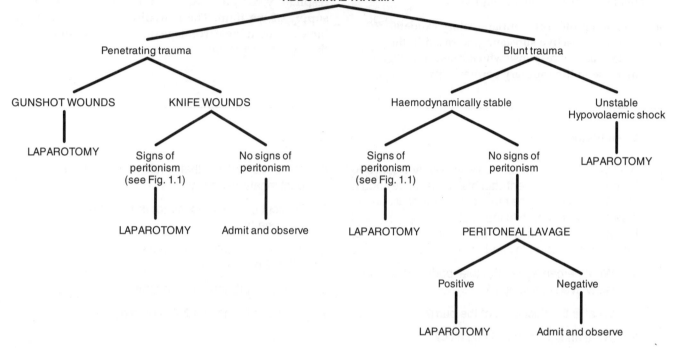

ABDOMINAL TRAUMA

Penetrating trauma

GUNSHOT WOUNDS → LAPAROTOMY

KNIFE WOUNDS
- Signs of peritonism (see Fig. 1.1) → LAPAROTOMY
- No signs of peritonism → Admit and observe

Blunt trauma

Haemodynamically stable
- Signs of peritonism (see Fig. 1.1) → LAPAROTOMY
- No signs of peritonism → PERITONEAL LAVAGE
  - Positive → LAPAROTOMY
  - Negative → Admit and observe

Unstable
Hypovolaemic shock → LAPAROTOMY

INTRODUCTION

A burn causes a loss of epidermis. This removes the barrier which prevents evaporation of body water. There is therefore a loss of fluid, the volume of which depends on the area of the burn.

This loss is further increased by:

a. loss of a protein-rich inflammatory exudate
b. loss of vasoactive substances released in the inflammatory response which cause a further increase in the capillary permeability

Loss of epidermis and the presence of necrotic tissue increase the likelihood of infection in a burn. A circumferential burn around the chest or a limb is called an *eschar* and risks limitation of chest expansion and hence respiratory compromise, or compromises the vascular supply of the limb. The mortality induced by a burn increases with the percentage of surface area burnt and the age of the patient.

Case history

A 32-year-old 74 kg man presents to an Accident and Emergency Department after his clothes have caught fire. On examination he has a circumferential burn on his left leg and a burn to the back of his right leg and buttock extending halfway up his back. The skin of the burn is white, shiny and anaesthetic.

1. What percentage of the total body surface area is involved in this burn?

2. What is the thickness of the burn?

3. What analgesia would you give?

4. List three findings that would make you suspect inhalation injury

5. Prescribe a fluid regime for the first 24 hours after the burn

7 hours after the burn the patient has produced a total of 175 ml of urine.

6. Is this a sufficient urine output?

7. Do these burns need skin grafting?

23.1 INITIAL ASSESSMENT

CLINICAL FEATURES
ASSESS SITE AND DEPTH OF BURN

FIRST-DEGREE BURNS
Erythema on burn site

SECOND-DEGREE/PARTIAL-THICKNESS BURNS
Vesicles, swelling and moist surface
Very painful

THIRD-DEGREE BURNS
Charred/waxen look
White or grey
Anaesthetic

PERCENTAGE OF
TOTAL BODY SURFACE AREA BURNT
Calculate by the rule of 9s:
– Head 9%
– Trunk 18% front, 18% back
– Arms 9% each
– Legs 18% each
– PALM IS 1% OF TOTAL

First- or second-degree, partial-thickness burns
affecting < 15% of total body surface area in adults
(< 10% in children)

May be treated as an outpatient

All full-thickness or third-degree burns
and first- or second-degree, partial-thickness burns
affecting > 15% of total body surface area in adults
(> 10% in children)

SITE OF BURN: Burns to:
– Hand – Face – Feet – Perineum
Circumferential burns to a limb

RESPIRATORY BURN: Suspicion of inhalation of hot gas or smoke
History of being caught in a smoky room
Facial skin burnt
Soot in the mouth
Burnt nasal hair

AGENT OF BURN: Electrical burn

**ABSOLUTE REQUIREMENT
FOR ADMISSION**

→ 3.2

23. MANAGEMENT OF A BURNED PATIENT

23.2 BURNS REQUIRING ADMISSION

AIRWAY AND BREATHING

FEATURES OF RESPIRATORY BURN

No features of respiratory burn

Arterial blood gases
Chest X-ray
Carboxyhaemoglobin level – if elevated, suggests carbon monoxide poisoning

Hypoxia
Raised carboxyhaemoglobin level
Abnormal chest X-ray

Normal arterial blood gases
Normal chest X-ray
Normal carboxyhaemoglobin level

RESPIRATORY FUNCTION COMPROMISED
Intubate and ventilate

No respiratory compromise
Beware: effects of smoke inhalation
may be delayed by up to 24 hours

REPLACE FLUID LOSS

$$\text{Replacement volume (ml)} = \frac{\text{Body weight (kg)} \times \% \text{ burns}}{2} \text{(colloid)}$$

Give this volume over each of three 4-hour periods,
the first calculated STARTING FROM TIME OF BURN
Same volume over next two 6-hour periods
Same volume over next 12 hours

Maintain urine output at >30ml/h

Tetanus prophylaxis

ANALGESIA – Intravenous opiates

ESCHAROTOMY
Circumferential burns of the limb may cause distal ischaemia
– and on the trunk they may cause respiratory embarassment
If necessary, divide them

CLEAN AND DEBRIDE BURN

PARTIAL-THICKNESS

Asepsis
Non-stick dressing

Re-epithelialize within 14–21 days

Infection may turn a partial-thickness burn to full-thickness

FULL-THICKNESS

Topical antibiotics
Remove dead skin

Graft priority areas first: hands, face and functional areas,
e.g. axilla, antecubital fossa
May use mesh grafts to gain more coverage

Pressure garments minimize hypertrophic scarring

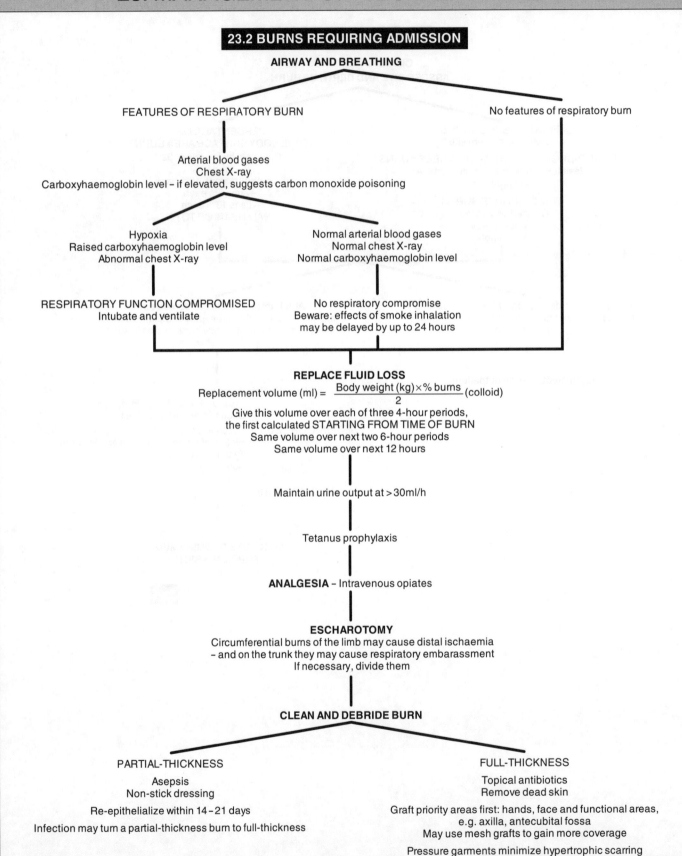

SECTION D

EAR, NOSE AND THROAT

This is predominantly a postgraduate subject. The aim of this section is to enable students to make a working diagnosis and intelligent referral to the specialist. The subjects covered in this section include:

1. Lumps in the neck
2. Epistaxis
3. Hoarse voice
4. Otalgia
5. Deafness

Examination of the ear includes:

a. *Inspection of the pinna*
b. *Inspection of the external auditory canal and tympanic membrane* using an auroscope
c. *Rinne's and Weber's tests*. Rinne's test compares air and bone conduction of sound through the middle ear. A tuning fork is sounded, placed near the ear and then directly over the mastoid process; the patient then indicates which sound is louder. If air conduction is better than bone conduction, the middle ear is functioning normally: Rinne-positive. If bone conduction is better than air conduction the middle ear is not functioning normally: Rinne-negative. In Weber's test the base of a tuning fork is placed on the forehead and the patient indicates the ear in which the sound is heard loudest. It is normally heard equally. In conductive deafness the sound is heard in the deafer ear; in sensorineural deafness the sound is heard in the good ear.

d. *Audiometry*. This measures hearing levels via air and bone conduction from 125 Hz to 12 000 Hz at variable intensities. Sounds of increasing intensity are used until the patient can hear the noise. A difference in the intensity heard between air and bone conduction – an 'air–bone gap' – indicates a conductive hearing loss.

e. *A tympanogram* tests the mobility of the tympanic membrane. It produces a flat trace in conditions that result in a loss of compliance of this membrane.

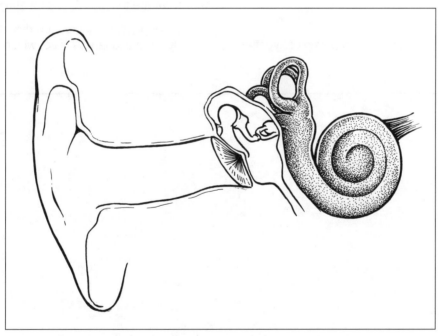

A defect in the shaded area causes a sensory neural deafness; in the plain area it causes a conductive deafness

24. LUMPS IN THE NECK

INTRODUCTION

Lumps in the neck are common and patients with lumps in the neck frequently appear in the clinical part of examinations. There are many structures in the neck which may enlarge and a knowledge of their sites and the frequency with which they enlarge is essential.

These lumps are best examined with the patient sitting down. Do not forget to examine the whole of the scalp, the back of the neck, the ears and the mouth and pharynx.

Case history

A 42-year-old lady presents with a swelling in her neck. This has been present for 5 months and is progressively enlarging. She is otherwise well. The lump is in the midline and moves on swallowing.

1. What two structures may cause this lump?

2. How would you differentiate them?

This lump moves only on swallowing, not on protruding the tongue. On palpation there is a regular smooth enlargement of the whole of the thyroid gland.

3. List four ophthalmic signs of hyperthyroidism.

4. What are the signs and symptoms of hypothyroidism?

5. What investigations would you do next?

This patient's thyroid function tests reveal low free thyroxine T4 and high TSH values.

6. Does this support a diagnosis of hypothyroidism or hyperthyroidism?

Anti-thyroid antibodies are present.

7. What is the diagnosis?

8. How would you further manage this patient?

9. What are the indications for surgery?

10. Is this patient at increased risk of developing a thyroid malignancy? If so, which type?

24. LUMPS IN THE NECK

24.1 INITIAL ASSESSMENT

Not in or around midline

In or around midline

Doesn't move on swallowing

Rarer differential diagnoses

Ranula
Dermoid cyst

Moves on swallowing

THYROID OR THYROGLOSSAL STRUCTURE → **24.6**

LOCATION
Locate the lump to one of the following regions:

Triangle between midline, anterior border of sternocleidomastoid and lower border of mandible

Triangle between posterior border of sternocleidomastoid and anterior border of trapezius and clavicle

Area bounded by zygoma superiorly, anteriorly over approximately one-third of masseter, posteriorly by mastoid process, inferiorly by stylomandibular ligament

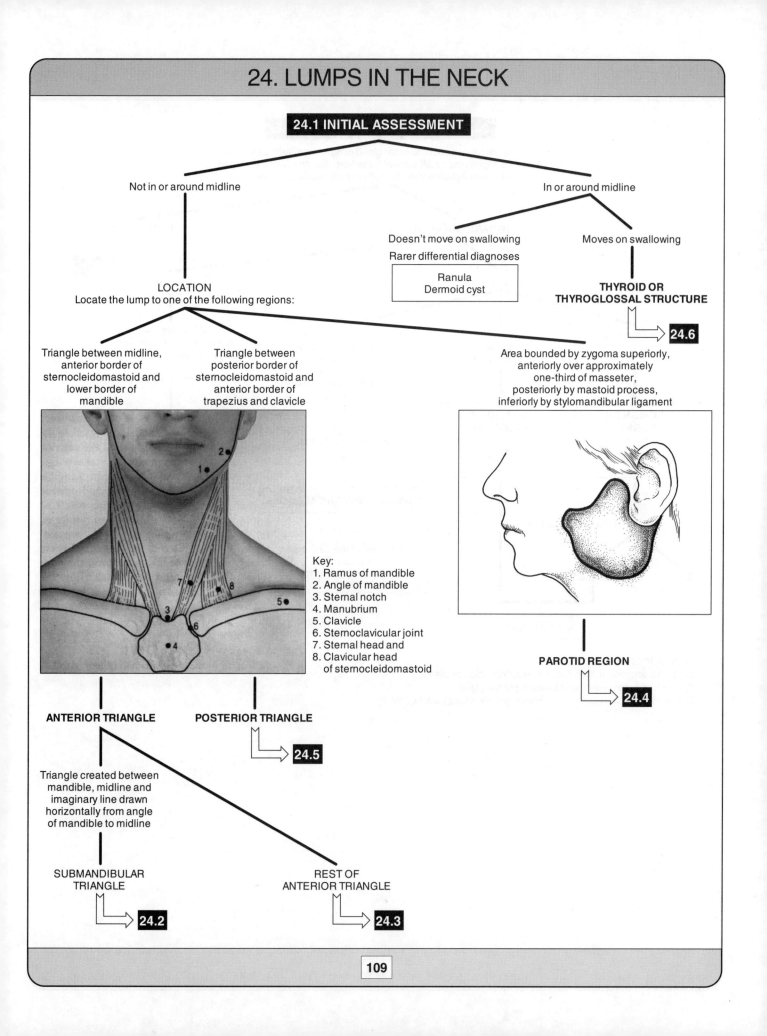

Key:
1. Ramus of mandible
2. Angle of mandible
3. Sternal notch
4. Manubrium
5. Clavicle
6. Sternoclavicular joint
7. Sternal head and
8. Clavicular head of sternocleidomastoid

PAROTID REGION → **24.4**

ANTERIOR TRIANGLE

POSTERIOR TRIANGLE → **24.5**

Triangle created between mandible, midline and imaginary line drawn horizontally from angle of mandible to midline

SUBMANDIBULAR TRIANGLE → **24.2**

REST OF ANTERIOR TRIANGLE → **24.3**

24.2 SUBMANDIBULAR TRIANGLE

Contents are either submandibular gland or submandibular lymph node
It may be impossible to differentiate one from the other when enlarged
Differentiation is therefore often made peroperatively

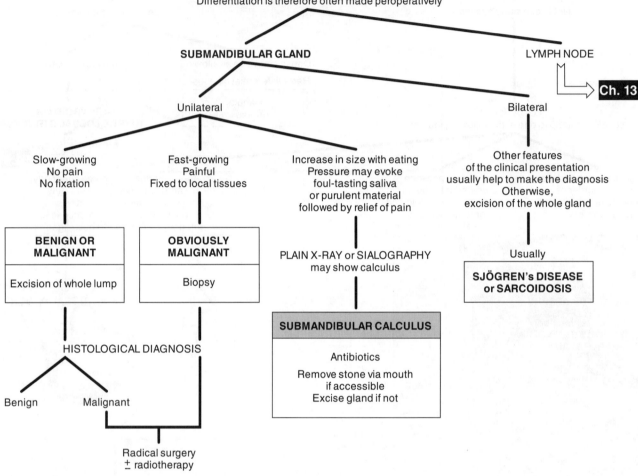

SUBMANDIBULAR GLAND

LYMPH NODE

Ch. 13

Unilateral

Bilateral

Slow-growing
No pain
No fixation

Fast-growing
Painful
Fixed to local tissues

Increase in size with eating
Pressure may evoke
foul-tasting saliva
or purulent material
followed by relief of pain

Other features
of the clinical presentation
usually help to make the diagnosis
Otherwise,
excision of the whole gland

BENIGN OR MALIGNANT	**OBVIOUSLY MALIGNANT**
Excision of whole lump	Biopsy

PLAIN X-RAY or SIALOGRAPHY
may show calculus

Usually

SJÖGREN's DISEASE or SARCOIDOSIS

HISTOLOGICAL DIAGNOSIS

Benign   Malignant

SUBMANDIBULAR CALCULUS
Antibiotics
Remove stone via mouth if accessible
Excise gland if not

Radical surgery
± radiotherapy

Some principles:
1. Stones commoner than tumours in submandibular gland
2. Tumours commoner than stones in parotid gland
3. The common tumours of both glands are the same (see Fig. 24.4)

24. LUMPS IN THE NECK

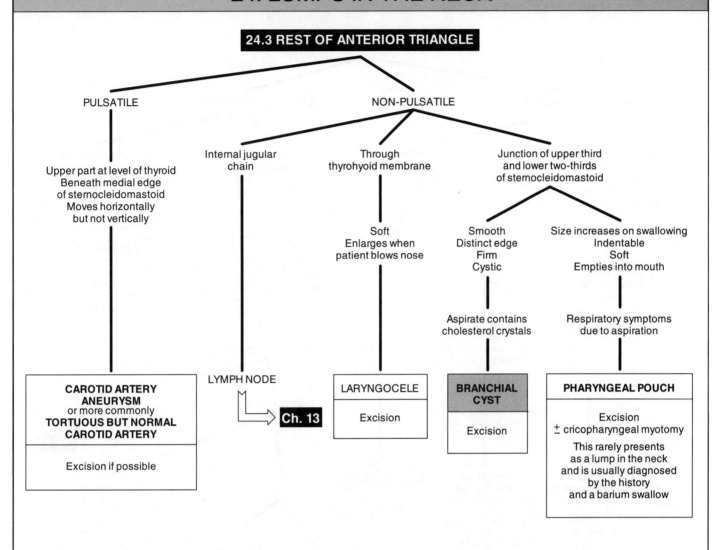

24.3 REST OF ANTERIOR TRIANGLE

PULSATILE

Upper part at level of thyroid
Beneath medial edge
of sternocleidomastoid
Moves horizontally
but not vertically

**CAROTID ARTERY
ANEURYSM**
or more commonly
**TORTUOUS BUT NORMAL
CAROTID ARTERY**

Excision if possible

NON-PULSATILE

Internal jugular chain

LYMPH NODE → **Ch. 13**

Through thyrohyoid membrane

Soft
Enlarges when
patient blows nose

LARYNGOCELE

Excision

Junction of upper third
and lower two-thirds
of sternocleidomastoid

Smooth
Distinct edge
Firm
Cystic

Aspirate contains
cholesterol crystals

**BRANCHIAL
CYST**

Excision

Size increases on swallowing
Indentable
Soft
Empties into mouth

Respiratory symptoms
due to aspiration

PHARYNGEAL POUCH

Excision
± cricopharyngeal myotomy

This rarely presents
as a lump in the neck
and is usually diagnosed
by the history
and a barium swallow

24. LUMPS IN THE NECK

24.4 PAROTID REGION

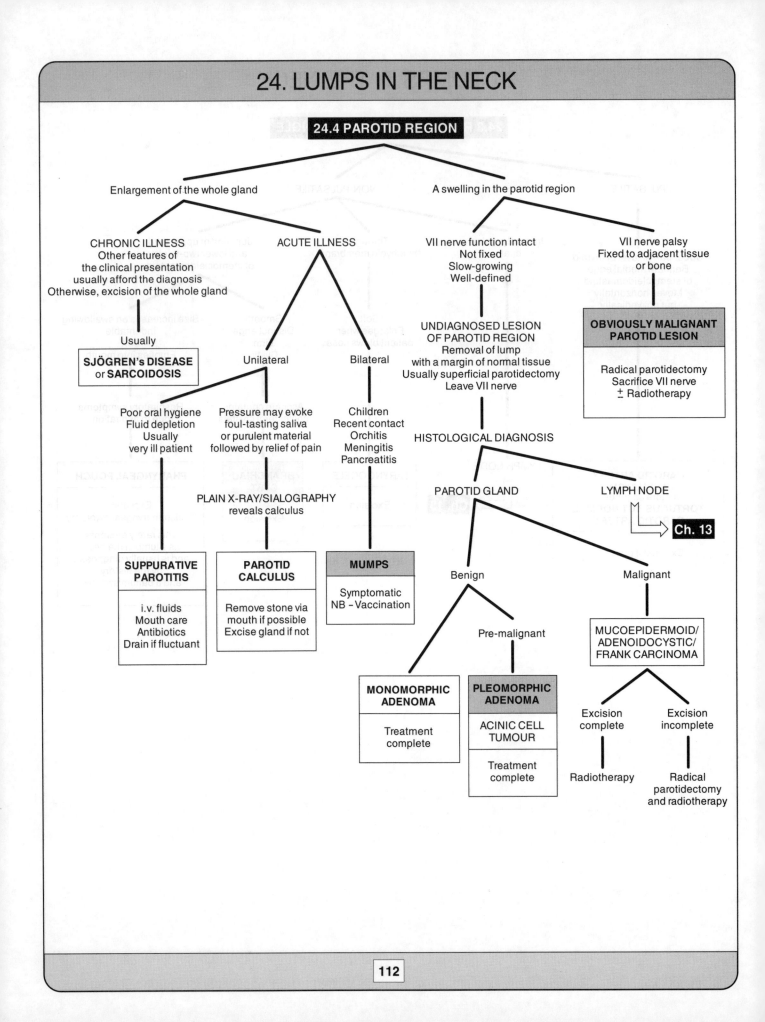

Enlargement of the whole gland

CHRONIC ILLNESS
Other features of
the clinical presentation
usually afford the diagnosis
Otherwise, excision of the whole gland

Usually

**SJÖGREN's DISEASE
or SARCOIDOSIS**

ACUTE ILLNESS

Unilateral

Poor oral hygiene
Fluid depletion
Usually
very ill patient

Pressure may evoke
foul-tasting saliva
or purulent material
followed by relief of pain

PLAIN X-RAY/SIALOGRAPHY
reveals calculus

Bilateral

Children
Recent contact
Orchitis
Meningitis
Pancreatitis

**SUPPURATIVE
PAROTITIS**

i.v. fluids
Mouth care
Antibiotics
Drain if fluctuant

**PAROTID
CALCULUS**

Remove stone via
mouth if possible
Excise gland if not

MUMPS

Symptomatic
NB – Vaccination

A swelling in the parotid region

VII nerve function intact
Not fixed
Slow-growing
Well-defined

**UNDIAGNOSED LESION
OF PAROTID REGION**
Removal of lump
with a margin of normal tissue
Usually superficial parotidectomy
Leave VII nerve

HISTOLOGICAL DIAGNOSIS

PAROTID GLAND

LYMPH NODE

Ch. 13

Benign

Malignant

Pre-malignant

**MONOMORPHIC
ADENOMA**

Treatment
complete

**PLEOMORPHIC
ADENOMA**

ACINIC CELL
TUMOUR

Treatment
complete

**MUCOEPIDERMOID/
ADENOIDOCYSTIC/
FRANK CARCINOMA**

Excision
complete

Radiotherapy

Excision
incomplete

Radical
parotidectomy
and radiotherapy

VII nerve palsy
Fixed to adjacent tissue
or bone

**OBVIOUSLY MALIGNANT
PAROTID LESION**

Radical parotidectomy
Sacrifice VII nerve
± Radiotherapy

24. LUMPS IN THE NECK

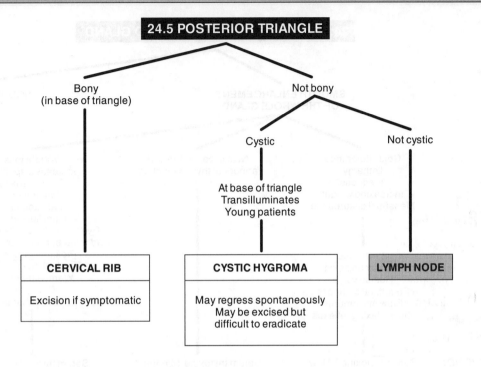

24.5 POSTERIOR TRIANGLE

Bony
(in base of triangle)

Not bony

Cystic

Not cystic

At base of triangle
Transilluminates
Young patients

CERVICAL RIB

Excision if symptomatic

CYSTIC HYGROMA

May regress spontaneously
May be excised but
difficult to eradicate

LYMPH NODE

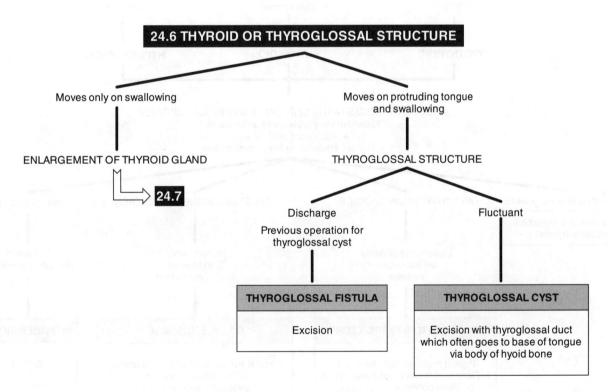

24.6 THYROID OR THYROGLOSSAL STRUCTURE

Moves only on swallowing

Moves on protruding tongue
and swallowing

ENLARGEMENT OF THYROID GLAND

→ 24.7

THYROGLOSSAL STRUCTURE

Discharge
Previous operation for
thyroglossal cyst

Fluctuant

THYROGLOSSAL FISTULA

Excision

THYROGLOSSAL CYST

Excision with thyroglossal duct
which often goes to base of tongue
via body of hyoid bone

24. LUMPS IN THE NECK

24.7 ENLARGEMENT OF THYROID GLAND

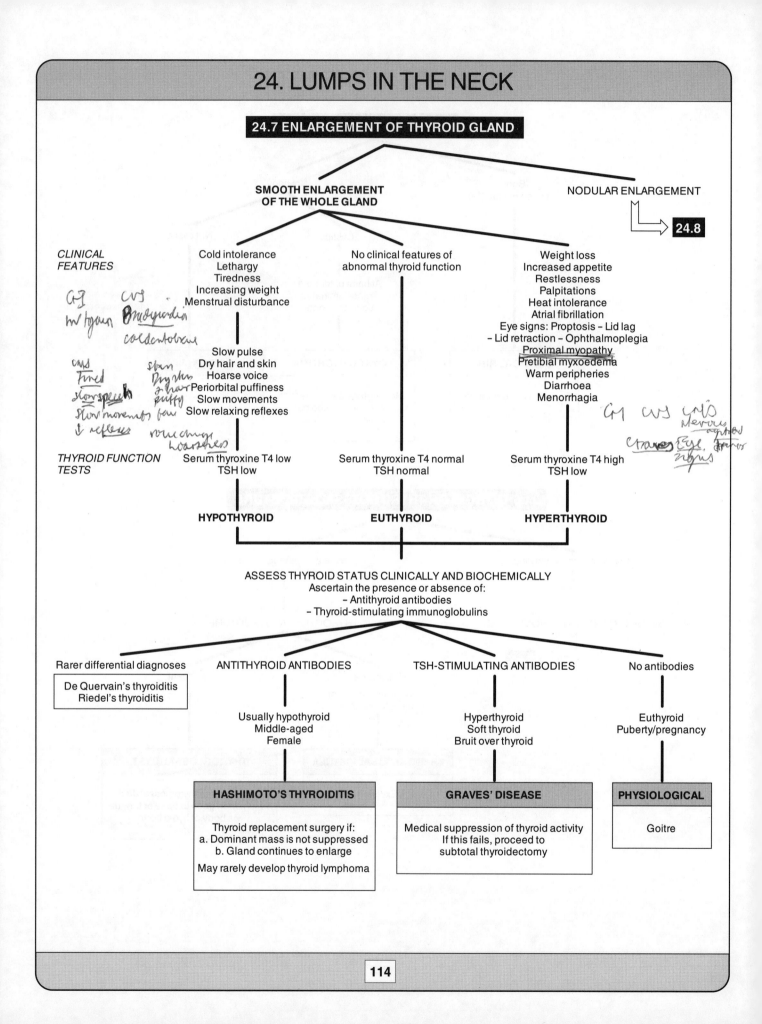

SMOOTH ENLARGEMENT OF THE WHOLE GLAND

NODULAR ENLARGEMENT → 24.8

CLINICAL FEATURES

Cold intolerance
Lethargy
Tiredness
Increasing weight
Menstrual disturbance

No clinical features of abnormal thyroid function

Weight loss
Increased appetite
Restlessness
Palpitations
Heat intolerance
Atrial fibrillation
Eye signs: Proptosis – Lid lag
– Lid retraction – Ophthalmoplegia
Proximal myopathy
Pretibial myxoedema
Warm peripheries
Diarrhoea
Menorrhagia

Slow pulse
Dry hair and skin
Hoarse voice
Periorbital puffiness
Slow movements
Slow relaxing reflexes

THYROID FUNCTION TESTS

Serum thyroxine T4 low
TSH low

Serum thyroxine T4 normal
TSH normal

Serum thyroxine T4 high
TSH low

HYPOTHYROID

EUTHYROID

HYPERTHYROID

ASSESS THYROID STATUS CLINICALLY AND BIOCHEMICALLY
Ascertain the presence or absence of:
– Antithyroid antibodies
– Thyroid-stimulating immunoglobulins

Rarer differential diagnoses

De Quervain's thyroiditis
Riedel's thyroiditis

ANTITHYROID ANTIBODIES

Usually hypothyroid
Middle-aged
Female

TSH-STIMULATING ANTIBODIES

Hyperthyroid
Soft thyroid
Bruit over thyroid

No antibodies

Euthyroid
Puberty/pregnancy

HASHIMOTO'S THYROIDITIS

Thyroid replacement surgery if:
a. Dominant mass is not suppressed
b. Gland continues to enlarge

May rarely develop thyroid lymphoma

GRAVES' DISEASE

Medical suppression of thyroid activity
If this fails, proceed to
subtotal thyroidectomy

PHYSIOLOGICAL

Goitre

24. LUMPS IN THE NECK

24.8 NODULAR ENLARGEMENT

SOLITARY NODULE

ULTRASOUND
Thyroid function tests → 40% of clinically solitary nodules are actually multiple → **MULTIPLE NODULES**

Confirms solitary nodule

Cystic

Solid

IODINE (^{131}I) RADIOISOTOPE SCAN

Doesn't take up radioisotope
TISSUE 'COLD' NODULE

Takes up radioisotope
TISSUE 'HOT' NODULE

FINE NEEDLE ASPIRATION CYTOLOGY
Otherwise **THYROID LOBECTOMY**

FUNCTIONING ADENOMA

Excision

THYROID CYST

Usually part of a multinodular goitre

Excision

Histology

Benign

Malignant

INACTIVE ADENOMATOUS NODULE

Excision

COLLOID NODULE

Excision

CARCINOMA

MALIGNANT LYMPHOMA OF THE THYROID

Resection and chemotherapy

Slow-growing
Non-invasive
Regular bosselated nodules

Recently enlarging
Invading adjacent tissues

Biopsy

MULTINODULAR GOITRE

To control thyrotoxicosis:
Antithyroid drugs
Radio-iodine ablation

Operation for:
– cosmesis
– tracheal or oesophageal compression

ANAPLASTIC CARCINOMA

Excision
if possible

PAPILLARY	**FOLLICULAR**	**ANAPLASTIC**	**MEDULLARY**
Commonest of thyroid malignancies Second and third decade Lymphatic spread Metastasise late	Middle-aged Metastasize late Blood spread	Elderly Local compressive and infiltrative symptoms Fixed to local tissues	Serum calcitonin raised
Total lobectomy/thyroidectomy with lymph node removal if obviously involved Thyroxine replacement therapy to suppress TSH	Total thyroidectomy and radio-iodine to metastases which take up iodine	Excision if possible Poor prognosis	Excision Screen family members by calcitonin, PTH and urinary catecholamine measurements for MENII

25. EPISTAXIS

INTRODUCTION

Expistaxis (nose bleeds) are common and usually trivial. In the rare life-threatening case it is important to resuscitate the patient by replacing the lost blood volume before trying to stop the bleeding.

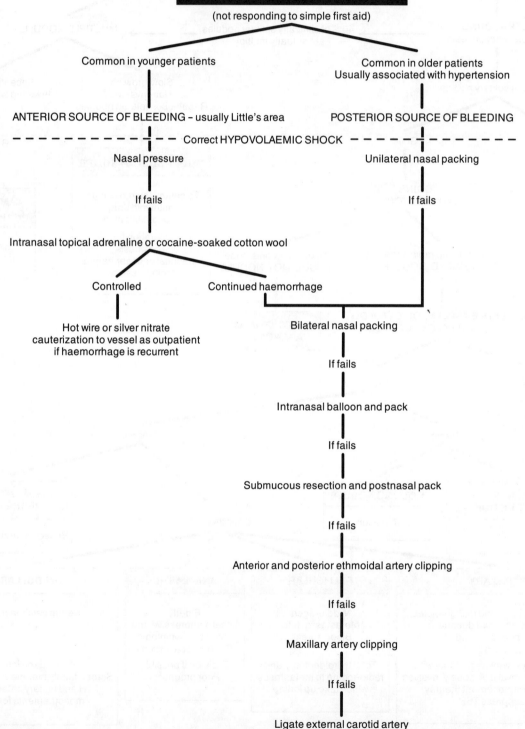

25.1 MANAGEMENT OF EPISTAXIS
(not responding to simple first aid)

Common in younger patients

Common in older patients
Usually associated with hypertension

ANTERIOR SOURCE OF BLEEDING – usually Little's area

POSTERIOR SOURCE OF BLEEDING

Correct HYPOVOLAEMIC SHOCK

Nasal pressure

Unilateral nasal packing

If fails

If fails

Intranasal topical adrenaline or cocaine-soaked cotton wool

Controlled

Continued haemorrhage

Hot wire or silver nitrate
cauterization to vessel as outpatient
if haemorrhage is recurrent

Bilateral nasal packing

If fails

Intranasal balloon and pack

If fails

Submucous resection and postnasal pack

If fails

Anterior and posterior ethmoidal artery clipping

If fails

Maxillary artery clipping

If fails

Ligate external carotid artery

26. HOARSE VOICE

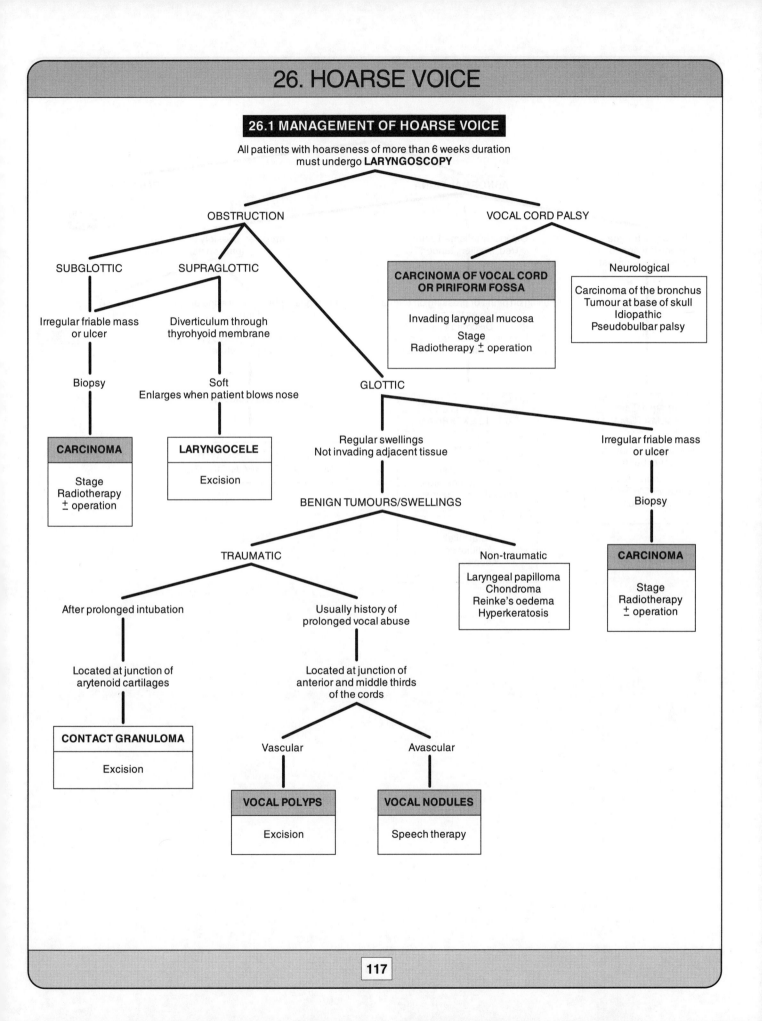

26.1 MANAGEMENT OF HOARSE VOICE

All patients with hoarseness of more than 6 weeks duration
must undergo **LARYNGOSCOPY**

OBSTRUCTION

VOCAL CORD PALSY

SUBGLOTTIC

SUPRAGLOTTIC

**CARCINOMA OF VOCAL CORD
OR PIRIFORM FOSSA**

Invading laryngeal mucosa

Stage
Radiotherapy ± operation

Neurological

Carcinoma of the bronchus
Tumour at base of skull
Idiopathic
Pseudobulbar palsy

Irregular friable mass
or ulcer

Diverticulum through
thyrohyoid membrane

Biopsy

Soft
Enlarges when patient blows nose

GLOTTIC

CARCINOMA

Stage
Radiotherapy
± operation

LARYNGOCELE

Excision

Regular swellings
Not invading adjacent tissue

Irregular friable mass
or ulcer

Biopsy

BENIGN TUMOURS/SWELLINGS

CARCINOMA

Stage
Radiotherapy
± operation

TRAUMATIC

Non-traumatic

Laryngeal papilloma
Chondroma
Reinke's oedema
Hyperkeratosis

After prolonged intubation

Usually history of
prolonged vocal abuse

Located at junction of
arytenoid cartilages

Located at junction of
anterior and middle thirds
of the cords

CONTACT GRANULOMA

Excision

Vascular

Avascular

VOCAL POLYPS

Excision

VOCAL NODULES

Speech therapy

27. OTALGIA

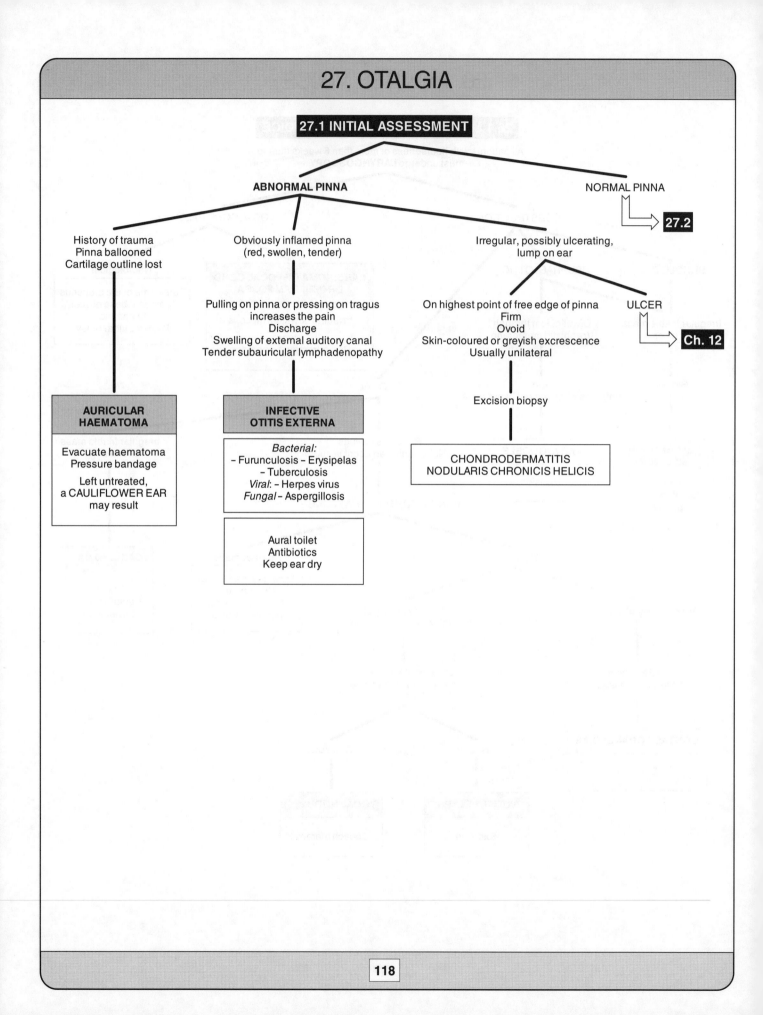

27.1 INITIAL ASSESSMENT

ABNORMAL PINNA

NORMAL PINNA → **27.2**

History of trauma
Pinna ballooned
Cartilage outline lost

Obviously inflamed pinna
(red, swollen, tender)

Irregular, possibly ulcerating, lump on ear

Pulling on pinna or pressing on tragus
increases the pain
Discharge
Swelling of external auditory canal
Tender subauricular lymphadenopathy

On highest point of free edge of pinna
Firm
Ovoid
Skin-coloured or greyish excrescence
Usually unilateral

ULCER → **Ch. 12**

Excision biopsy

AURICULAR HAEMATOMA

Evacuate haematoma
Pressure bandage

Left untreated,
a CAULIFLOWER EAR
may result

INFECTIVE OTITIS EXTERNA

Bacterial:
– Furunculosis – Erysipelas
– Tuberculosis
Viral: – Herpes virus
Fungal – Aspergillosis

Aural toilet
Antibiotics
Keep ear dry

CHONDRODERMATITIS
NODULARIS CHRONICIS HELICIS

27. OTALGIA

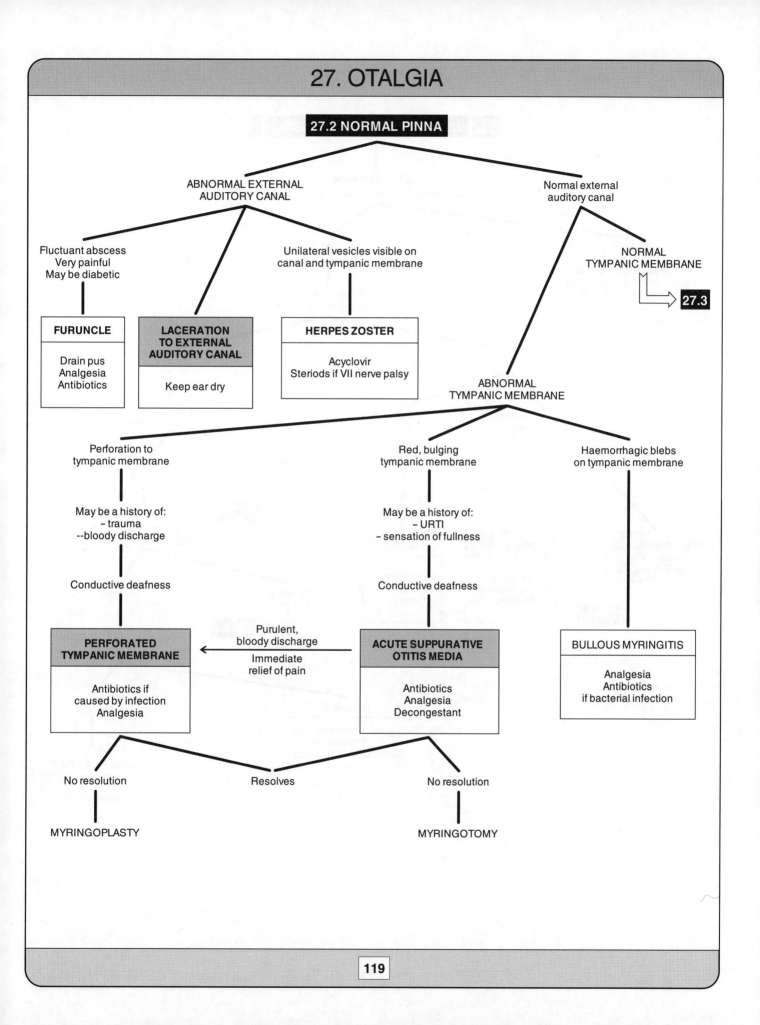

27.2 NORMAL PINNA

ABNORMAL EXTERNAL AUDITORY CANAL

Normal external auditory canal

Fluctuant abscess
Very painful
May be diabetic

Unilateral vesicles visible on canal and tympanic membrane

NORMAL TYMPANIC MEMBRANE

→ **27.3**

FURUNCLE

Drain pus
Analgesia
Antibiotics

LACERATION TO EXTERNAL AUDITORY CANAL

Keep ear dry

HERPES ZOSTER

Acyclovir
Steriods if VII nerve palsy

ABNORMAL TYMPANIC MEMBRANE

Perforation to tympanic membrane

Red, bulging tympanic membrane

Haemorrhagic blebs on tympanic membrane

May be a history of:
– trauma
--bloody discharge

May be a history of:
– URTI
– sensation of fullness

Conductive deafness

Conductive deafness

PERFORATED TYMPANIC MEMBRANE

Antibiotics if caused by infection
Analgesia

Purulent, bloody discharge
Immediate relief of pain

ACUTE SUPPURATIVE OTITIS MEDIA

Antibiotics
Analgesia
Decongestant

BULLOUS MYRINGITIS

Analgesia
Antibiotics
if bacterial infection

No resolution

Resolves

No resolution

MYRINGOPLASTY

MYRINGOTOMY

27. OTALGIA

27.3 NORMAL TYMPANIC MEMBRANE

REFERRED PAIN
Examination of teeth and mucosa of oral cavity

Abnormal

Infected or impacted teeth
Traumatic or malignant ulcer
Temperomandibular joint
dysfunction

Normal

Examination of
oropharynx and mouth

Abnormal

Pyrexia
Enlarged
hyperaemic tonsils
± Pus
± Fetor
Tender cervical
lymphadenopathy

Pyrexia
± Fetor
± Dysphagia

Peritonsillar abscess

**TRAUMATIC OR
MALIGNANT
ULCER**

→ Ch. 12

TONSILLITIS

Soluble aspirin
Encourage fluids
Antibiotics

QUINSY

i.v. antibiotics
± i.v. fluids
Drain pus

Normal

Examination of
larynx and pharynx

Abnormal

→ Ch. 26

Normal

Examination of
neck and skin of scalp

Abnormal

→ Ch. 24

Normal

Examination of nose,
postnasal space and sinuses

Abnormal

Carcinoma of postnasal space
Sinusitis
Carcinoma of the sinus

Normal

INNER EAR PAIN

Refer to specialist

120

28. DEAFNESS

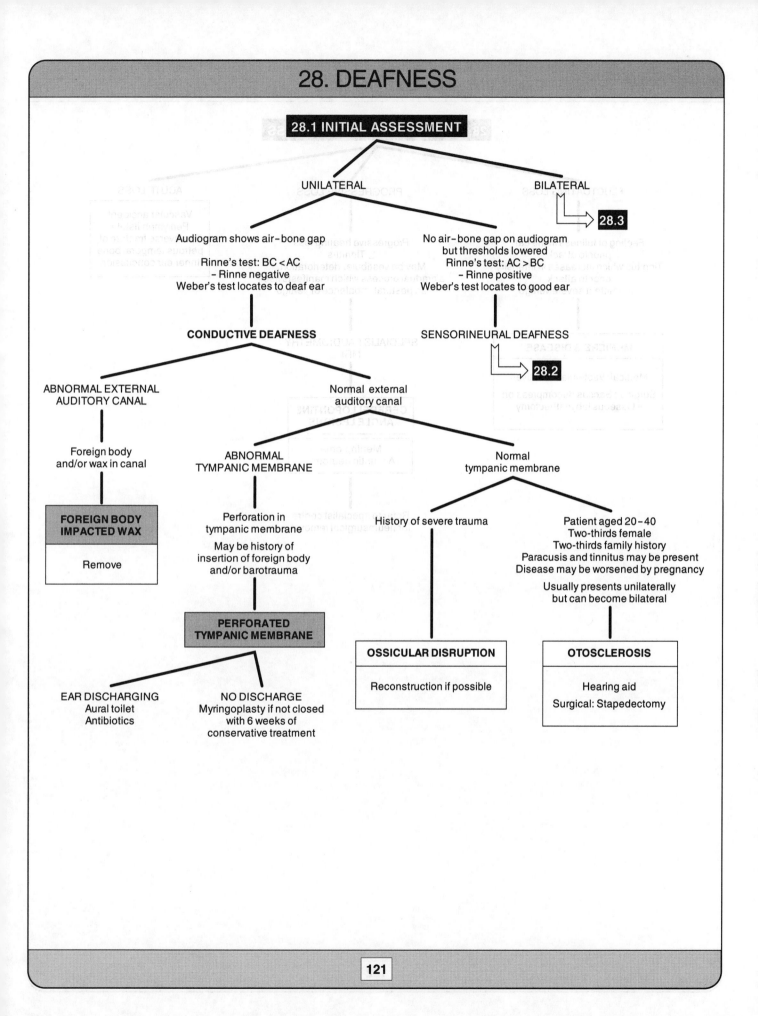

UNILATERAL

BILATERAL → **28.3**

Audiogram shows air–bone gap

Rinne's test: BC < AC
– Rinne negative
Weber's test locates to deaf ear

No air–bone gap on audiogram
but thresholds lowered
Rinne's test: AC > BC
– Rinne positive
Weber's test locates to good ear

CONDUCTIVE DEAFNESS

SENSORINEURAL DEAFNESS → **28.2**

ABNORMAL EXTERNAL
AUDITORY CANAL

Normal external
auditory canal

Foreign body
and/or wax in canal

ABNORMAL
TYMPANIC MEMBRANE

Normal
tympanic membrane

**FOREIGN BODY
IMPACTED WAX**

Remove

Perforation in
tympanic membrane

May be history of
insertion of foreign body
and/or barotrauma

History of severe trauma

Patient aged 20–40
Two-thirds female
Two-thirds family history
Paracusis and tinnitus may be present
Disease may be worsened by pregnancy

Usually presents unilaterally
but can become bilateral

**PERFORATED
TYMPANIC MEMBRANE**

OSSICULAR DISRUPTION

Reconstruction if possible

OTOSCLEROSIS

Hearing aid
Surgical: Stapedectomy

EAR DISCHARGING
Aural toilet
Antibiotics

NO DISCHARGE
Myringoplasty if not closed
with 6 weeks of
conservative treatment

28. DEAFNESS

28.2 SENSORINEURAL DEAFNESS

FLUCTUATING LOSS

Feeling of fullness in the ear
prior to attack
Tinnitus which increases in intensity
prior to attack
Intermittent severe vertigo

MENIÈRE'S DISEASE

Medical: Vestibular sedatives

Surgical: Saccus decompression
– Osseous labyrinthectomy

PROGRESSIVE LOSS

Progressive hearing loss
± Tinnitus
May be vestibular deterioration,
a gradual process which manifests itself
as postural imbalance or vertigo

SPECIALIST AUDIOMETRY
MRI

CEREBELLOPONTINE
ANGLE LESIONS

Meningioma
Acoustic neuroma

Refer to specialist centre
for neurosurgical removal

ACUTE LOSS

Vascular accident
Perilymph fistula
Transverse fracture of
petrous temporal bone
Inner ear concussion

28. DEAFNESS

28.3 BILATERAL DEAFNESS

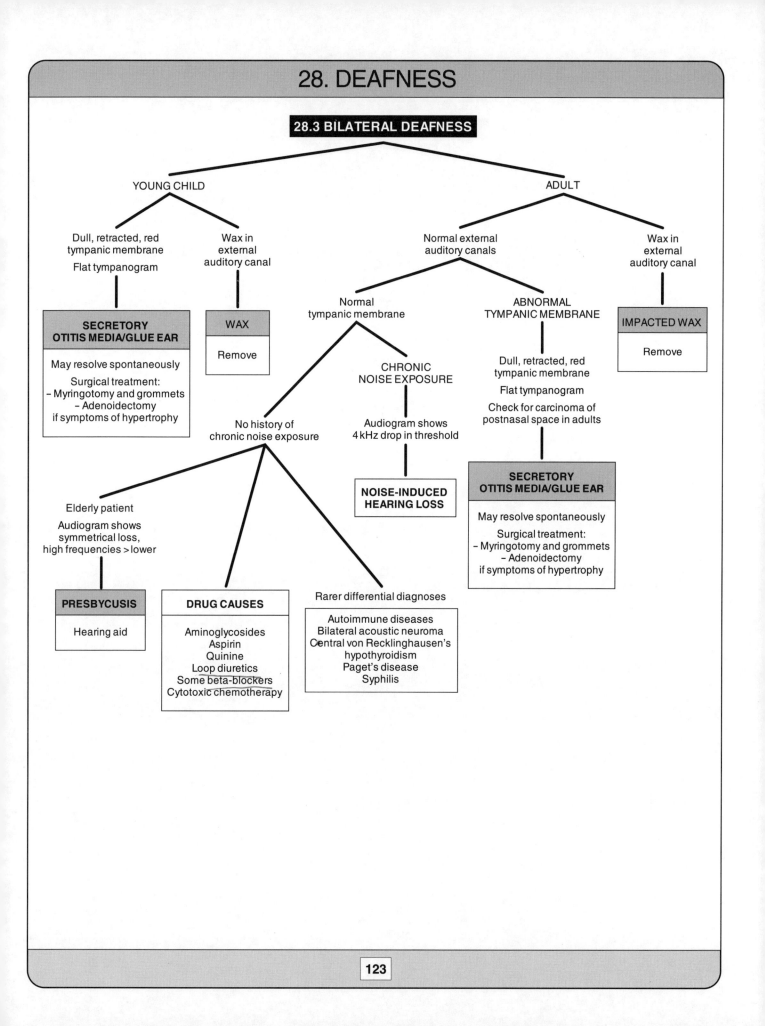

YOUNG CHILD

Dull, retracted, red tympanic membrane

Flat tympanogram

SECRETORY OTITIS MEDIA/GLUE EAR

May resolve spontaneously

Surgical treatment:
– Myringotomy and grommets
– Adenoidectomy
if symptoms of hypertrophy

Wax in external auditory canal

WAX

Remove

ADULT

Normal external auditory canals

Normal tympanic membrane

No history of chronic noise exposure

Elderly patient

Audiogram shows symmetrical loss, high frequencies > lower

PRESBYCUSIS

Hearing aid

DRUG CAUSES

Aminoglycosides
Aspirin
Quinine
Loop diuretics
Some beta-blockers
Cytotoxic chemotherapy

Rarer differential diagnoses

Autoimmune diseases
Bilateral acoustic neuroma
Central von Recklinghausen's
hypothyroidism
Paget's disease
Syphilis

CHRONIC NOISE EXPOSURE

Audiogram shows 4 kHz drop in threshold

NOISE-INDUCED HEARING LOSS

ABNORMAL TYMPANIC MEMBRANE

Dull, retracted, red tympanic membrane

Flat tympanogram

Check for carcinoma of postnasal space in adults

SECRETORY OTITIS MEDIA/GLUE EAR

May resolve spontaneously

Surgical treatment:
– Myringotomy and grommets
– Adenoidectomy
if symptoms of hypertrophy

Wax in external auditory canal

IMPACTED WAX

Remove

SECTION E

OPHTHALMOLOGY

INTRODUCTION

The management of eye disease is essentially a post-graduate subject. The aim of this chapter is to introduce the non-specialist to the assessment of basic ophthalmic presentations and equip him or her with the skills to make an intelligent referral to the specialist. The most common presentations seen by non-specialists are acute red eye and sudden painless loss of vision. These subjects will be addressed in Chapters 29 and 30 respectively.

The essential examination of an eye includes:

a. The measurement of visual acuity.

b. The assessment of the eye media (anterior chamber, lens, posterior chamber), based on examination with a slit lamp microscope and fluorescein, and the measurement of intraocular pressure by applanation tonometry.

c. The assessment of pupillary signs and the presence or absence of relative afferent pupillary defect (RAPD). This is a sign elicited by illuminating each eye in turn to the count of three. The pupils should maintain an equal constriction as the light source is moved across the bridge of the nose from one eye to the other. Persistent unilateral pupillary dilatation as the light source is moved back to that side denotes a relative afferent pupillary defect on that side.

d. The assessment of the optic disc and retina, examined with an ophthalmoscope.

In order to understand the principles of eye disease, a basic understanding of the anatomy is useful, as shown in the diagram below.

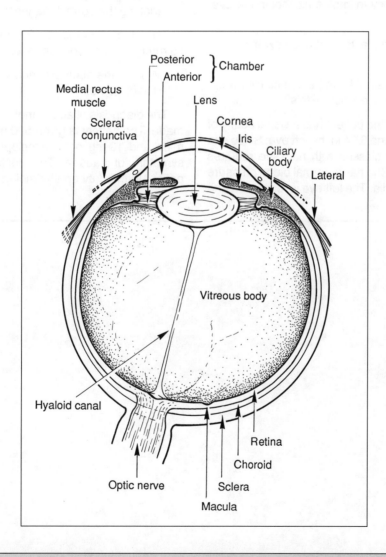

Case history

A 45-year-old diabetic woman with no previous history of eye trouble presents complaining of a painful, red left eye. They eye became acutely painful earlier in the afternoon, rendering her unable to continue her job as a machinist. Simple analgesia has had no effect. The patient admits to feeling nauseous and dizzy and has a 'terrible headache', but ascribes that to a hangover acquired the previous evening.

The casualty officer notes in the history that the patient's vision has deteriorated, particularly at night, with reduced field of vision, and lights are seen to be 'fuzzy'. Direct light hurts her eyes, and she complains of seeing 'rainbows' around light bulbs. She herself has ascribed this change in her vision to increasing age and her tendency to imbibe alcohol in the evenings.

1. What are the first facts to note on examination?

2. The patient does not have her spectacles with her; what is the relevance of this?

On examination, the patient has a visual acuity of 6/9 in the right eye and 6/24 in the left eye. Since she does not have her glasses with her, she requires pinhole correction. She has a normal blood pressure and sinus tachycardia. The left eye is tense, red and without obvious proptosis or conjunctival oedema. The right eye appears normal.

3. Given the detailed story of the character of the visual changes, what is the most likely diagnosis and what might the doctor expect to find on further examination of her eyes?

The left eye is mildly photophobic and the left pupil is dilated and slower to react than the normal right one. The corneas are asymmetrical, the left cloudier than the right. The anterior chambers are clear on both sides. Funduscopy reveals a normal right disc and the left is not seen.

4. What investigation is of paramount importance in making the correct diagnosis?

The doctor notes an intraocular pressure of 45 mmHg by applanation tonometry.

5. What is the diagnosis and what does the doctor do next?

The diagnosis of acute angle closure glaucoma is made. The patient is given 500 mg of i.v. acetazolamide and 10 mg oral metoclopramide to allay the symptom of nausea. The doctor then refers the patient to the duty ophthalmologist.

29. ACUTE RED EYE

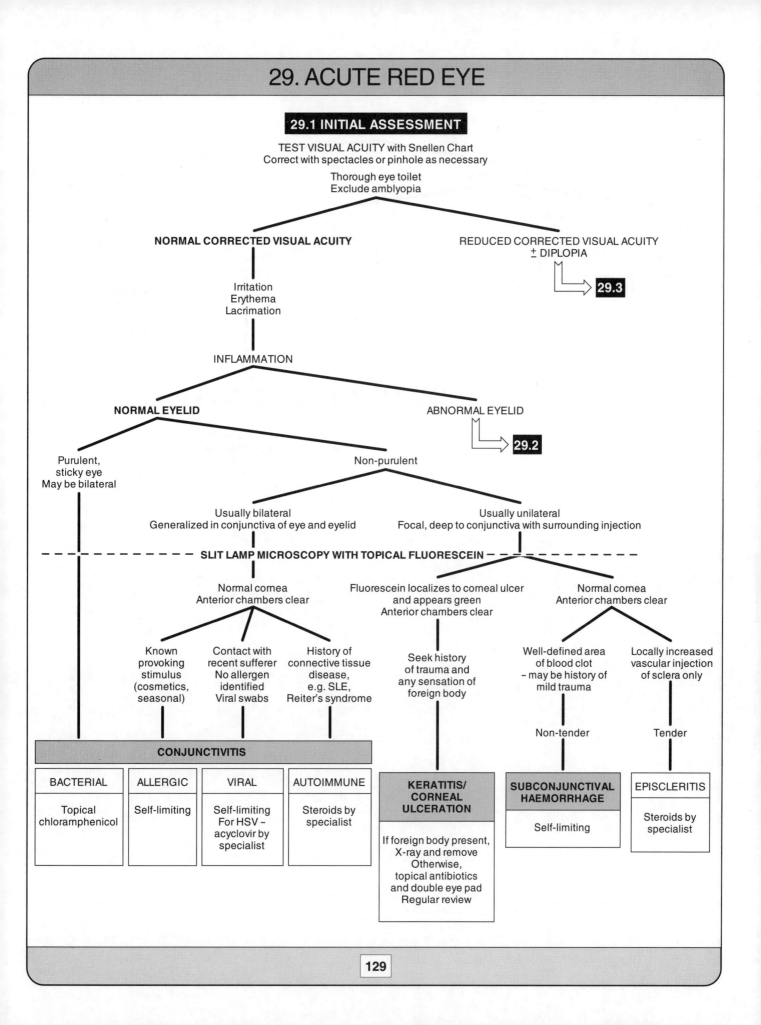

29.1 INITIAL ASSESSMENT

TEST VISUAL ACUITY with Snellen Chart
Correct with spectacles or pinhole as necessary

Thorough eye toilet
Exclude amblyopia

NORMAL CORRECTED VISUAL ACUITY

REDUCED CORRECTED VISUAL ACUITY ± DIPLOPIA → **29.3**

Irritation
Erythema
Lacrimation

INFLAMMATION

NORMAL EYELID

ABNORMAL EYELID → **29.2**

Purulent, sticky eye
May be bilateral

Non-purulent

Usually bilateral
Generalized in conjunctiva of eye and eyelid

Usually unilateral
Focal, deep to conjunctiva with surrounding injection

— — — — **SLIT LAMP MICROSCOPY WITH TOPICAL FLUORESCEIN** — — — —

Normal cornea
Anterior chambers clear

Fluorescein localizes to corneal ulcer and appears green
Anterior chambers clear

Normal cornea
Anterior chambers clear

Known provoking stimulus (cosmetics, seasonal)

Contact with recent sufferer
No allergen identified
Viral swabs

History of connective tissue disease, e.g. SLE, Reiter's syndrome

Seek history of trauma and any sensation of foreign body

Well-defined area of blood clot – may be history of mild trauma

Locally increased vascular injection of sclera only

Non-tender

Tender

CONJUNCTIVITIS

BACTERIAL	ALLERGIC	VIRAL	AUTOIMMUNE
Topical chloramphenicol	Self-limiting	Self-limiting For HSV – acyclovir by specialist	Steroids by specialist

KERATITIS/ CORNEAL ULCERATION

If foreign body present, X-ray and remove
Otherwise, topical antibiotics and double eye pad
Regular review

SUBCONJUNCTIVAL HAEMORRHAGE

Self-limiting

EPISCLERITIS

Steroids by specialist

29. ACUTE RED EYE

29.2 ABNORMAL EYELID

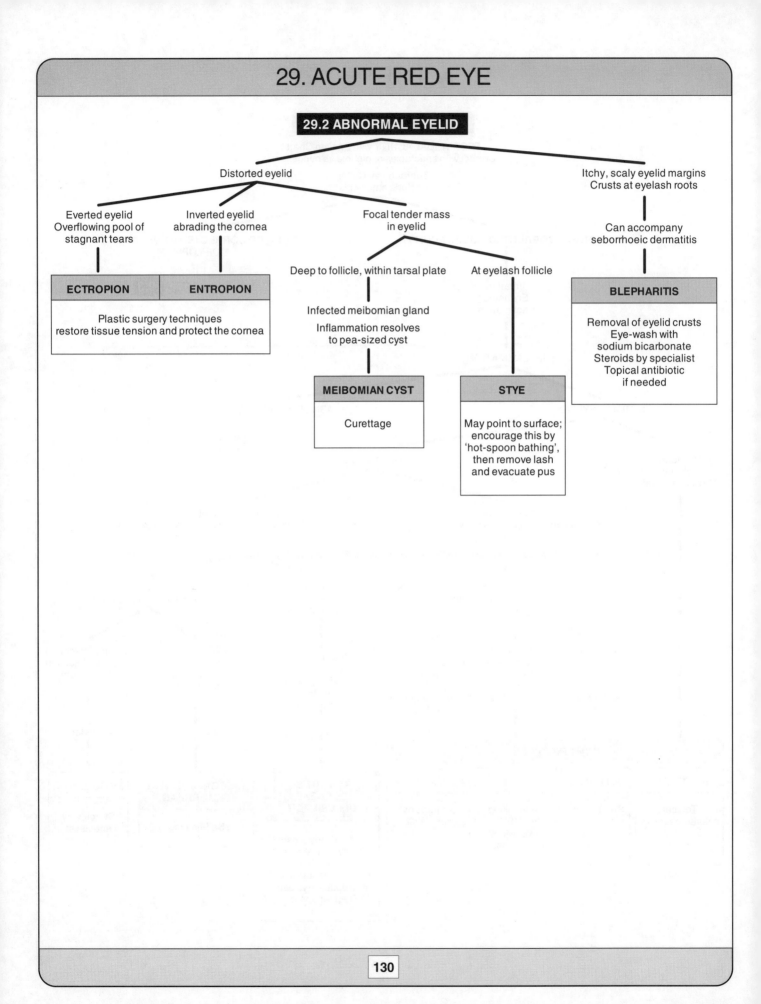

Distorted eyelid

Itchy, scaly eyelid margins
Crusts at eyelash roots

Everted eyelid
Overflowing pool of
stagnant tears

Inverted eyelid
abrading the cornea

Focal tender mass
in eyelid

Can accompany
seborrhoeic dermatitis

ECTROPION	ENTROPION
Plastic surgery techniques restore tissue tension and protect the cornea	

Deep to follicle, within tarsal plate

At eyelash follicle

Infected meibomian gland
Inflammation resolves
to pea-sized cyst

BLEPHARITIS

Removal of eyelid crusts
Eye-wash with
sodium bicarbonate
Steroids by specialist
Topical antibiotic
if needed

MEIBOMIAN CYST

Curettage

STYE

May point to surface;
encourage this by
'hot-spoon bathing',
then remove lash
and evacuate pus

29. ACUTE RED EYE

29.3 REDUCED CORRECTED VISUAL ACUITY

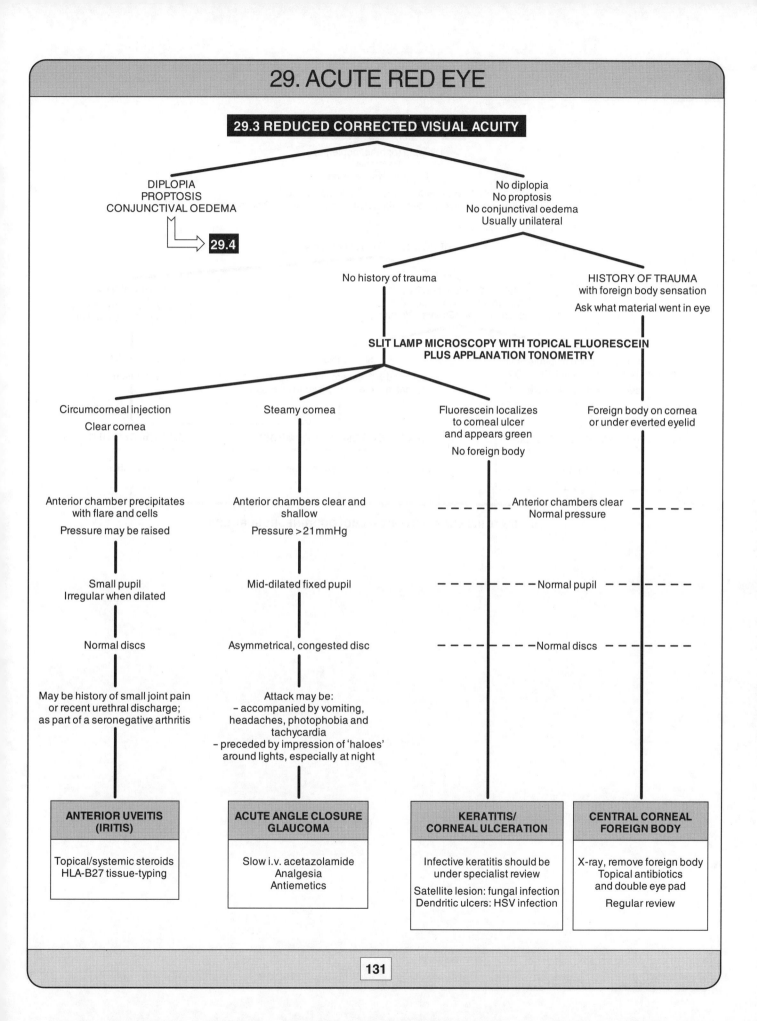

DIPLOPIA
PROPTOSIS
CONJUNCTIVAL OEDEMA

29.4

No diplopia
No proptosis
No conjunctival oedema
Usually unilateral

No history of trauma

HISTORY OF TRAUMA
with foreign body sensation

Ask what material went in eye

**SLIT LAMP MICROSCOPY WITH TOPICAL FLUORESCEIN
PLUS APPLANATION TONOMETRY**

Circumcorneal injection	Steamy cornea	Fluorescein localizes	Foreign body on cornea
Clear cornea		to corneal ulcer and appears green	or under everted eyelid
		No foreign body	

Anterior chamber precipitates
with flare and cells

Pressure may be raised

Anterior chambers clear and
shallow

Pressure >21 mmHg

Anterior chambers clear
Normal pressure

Small pupil
Irregular when dilated

Mid-dilated fixed pupil

Normal pupil

Normal discs

Asymmetrical, congested disc

Normal discs

May be history of small joint pain
or recent urethral discharge;
as part of a seronegative arthritis

Attack may be:
– accompanied by vomiting,
headaches, photophobia and
tachycardia
– preceded by impression of 'haloes'
around lights, especially at night

ANTERIOR UVEITIS (IRITIS)	**ACUTE ANGLE CLOSURE GLAUCOMA**	**KERATITIS/ CORNEAL ULCERATION**	**CENTRAL CORNEAL FOREIGN BODY**
Topical/systemic steroids HLA-B27 tissue-typing	Slow i.v. acetazolamide Analgesia Antiemetics	Infective keratitis should be under specialist review Satellite lesion: fungal infection Dendritic ulcers: HSV infection	X-ray, remove foreign body Topical antibiotics and double eye pad Regular review

29.4 RARE CONDITIONS

Diplopia (ophthalmoplegia)
Proptosis
Conjunctival oedema

These conditions are rare but very serious
They all have a range of presentations, which may be very subtle in nature

RESCUSCITATE as necessary

SIGNS OF MENINGISM:
– Photophobia – Neck stiffness
– Headache – Papilloedema – Vomiting

Not meningitic

Usually occurs in children
with intercurrent infection

Pulsatile proptosis with palpable thrill
and bruit synchronous with the pulse

Raised intraocular pressure

Non-pulsatile

Associated with severe intercurrent illness
or local (middle-ear/lip/sinus) infection

Eyelids difficult to open

Obvious inflammation

CAROTICOCAVERNOUS FISTULA
Resuscitate

CAVERNOUS SINUS THROMBOSIS
Resuscitate; antibiotics as appropriate

ORBITAL CELLULITIS
Antibiotics

IMMEDIATE REFERRAL TO OPHTHALMOLOGIST/NEUROSURGEON

30. SUDDEN PAINLESS LOSS OF VISION

30.1 INITIAL ASSESSMENT (1)

FIELD LOSS AFFECTING ONE EYE ONLY

FIELD LOSS AFFECTING BOTH EYES → **30.2**

Relative afferent pupillary defect (RAPD)
Media clear

No relative afferent pupillary defect (RAPD) → **30.2**

Severe loss of vision
i.e. see less than hand movements

Moderate loss of vision
i.e. see more than hand movements

Acute onset

Acute onset

Visual loss has slower onset,
over 1–2 days;
may begin with peripheral field loss

Normal retina

Oedematous white retina
Cherry-red spot in macula
(choroid shows through)

Retinal
'stormy sunset' picture:
superficial irregular
haemorrhages,
tortuous vessels and
arteriovenous nipping

Eye pain on movement,
with reduced colour vision
and episodic diplopia

Spots/flashes in vision,
or history of
curtains falling across
the visual field

Swollen,
haemorrhagic disc

Normal disc

Swollen,
haemorrhagic disc

Normal retina with
normal or swollen disc

Grey, opalescent retina
which balloons anteriorly
Normal disc

Delayed visual evoked
response (VER)
plus MRI evidence
of demyelination

Confirmed with
OCULAR ULTRASOUND

ANTERIOR ISCHAEMIC OPTIC NEUROPATHY	**RETINAL ARTERY OCCLUSION**	**RETINAL VEIN OCCLUSION**	**OPTIC NEURITIS**	**RETINAL DETACHMENT**
Profound and permanent visual loss. Urgent treatment involves firm ocular massage, i.v. acetazolamide and anterior chamber paracentesis to reduce ocular pressure. Must test ESR: – an elevated result with headaches, scalp tenderness, jaw claudication and girdle stiffness suggests GIANT CELL ARTERITIS. The patient is at risk of continued infarction and blindness if the diagnosis is missed. Confirm with temporal artery biopsy		Visual loss reflects degree of macular oedema and ischaemia. There is no treatment	May herald the onset of multiple sclerosis. Vision slowly recovers. Steroids may be of benefit	Cryotherapy, laser coagulation, ± vitrectomy

30. SUDDEN PAINLESS LOSS OF VISION

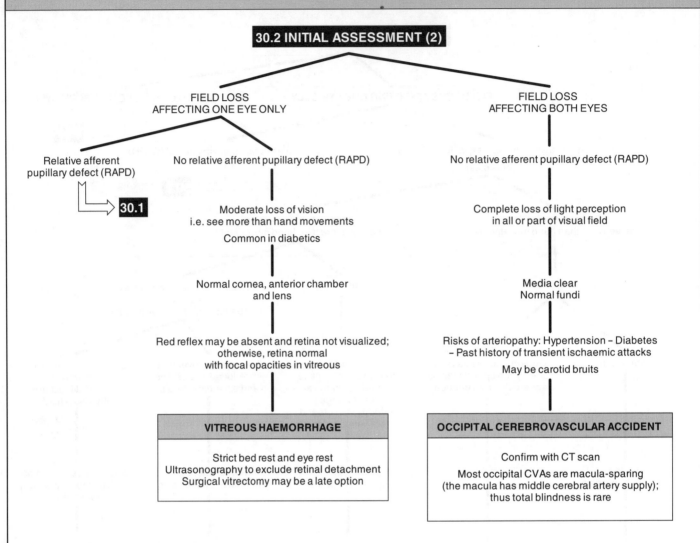

30.2 INITIAL ASSESSMENT (2)

FIELD LOSS AFFECTING ONE EYE ONLY

Relative afferent pupillary defect (RAPD)

→ 30.1

No relative afferent pupillary defect (RAPD)

Moderate loss of vision
i.e. see more than hand movements

Common in diabetics

Normal cornea, anterior chamber
and lens

Red reflex may be absent and retina not visualized;
otherwise, retina normal
with focal opacities in vitreous

VITREOUS HAEMORRHAGE

Strict bed rest and eye rest
Ultrasonography to exclude retinal detachment
Surgical vitrectomy may be a late option

FIELD LOSS AFFECTING BOTH EYES

No relative afferent pupillary defect (RAPD)

Complete loss of light perception
in all or part of visual field

Media clear
Normal fundi

Risks of arteriopathy: Hypertension – Diabetes
– Past history of transient ischaemic attacks

May be carotid bruits

OCCIPITAL CEREBROVASCULAR ACCIDENT

Confirm with CT scan

Most occipital CVAs are macula-sparing
(the macula has middle cerebral artery supply);
thus total blindness is rare

THE GLAUCOMAS

Glaucoma (characterized by a high intraocular pressure – IOP) are primarily described as open-angle or closed-angle, according to the mechanism of raised IOP. They may be primary or secondary (e.g. to new vessel formation in diabetes, or past trauma), congenital or adult-onset.

Primary closed-angle glaucoma occurs in anatomically predisposed eyes where aqueous outflow is obstructed by the peripheral iris. Designed to reduce IOP (often > 50 mmHg), the initial treatment is medical and the definitive procedures are surgical.

The first line of treatment is drugs which reduce production of the aqueous such as timolol and acetazolamide.

a. An intravenous loading dose of acetazolamide is followed by regular oral doses.
b. Pilocarpine (a miotic) is given when the reduction in IOP is sufficient to allow significant bloodstream perfusion.
c. Analgesia and antiemetics provide symptomatic relief.
d. Hyperosmotic drugs such as isosorbide and mannitol act to draw fluid out of the eye and reduce the IOP.

Later surgical options include peripheral iridectomy and laser iridotomy (often as outpatient local anaesthetic procedures) to increase aqueous drainage.

Primary open-angle glaucoma does not usually present as acute red eye. It is a condition of insidious onset which manifests itself as a significant loss of visual field and the diagnosis is made by serial IOP measurements and formal field testing.

ANTERIOR UVEITIS

The uveal tract includes the iris, ciliary body, choroid and retina. There are a number of causes of inflammation here (infective, granulomatous, autoimmune), including a collection of miscellaneous conditions. Only acute anterior uveal inflammation will result in acute red eye; in chronic conditions the eye may be white and asymptomatic though severely inflamed.

The majority of cases are part of a systemic inflammatory disease process, most commonly ankylosing spondylitis (including the group of seronegative HLA-B27-associated arthropathies) and multisystem sarcoidosis. They are managed jointly by ophthalmologists and physicians and anti-inflammatory steroids, administered topically, systemically and by periocular injection, are the mainstay of treatment. Rare but treatable causes include tuberculosis and syphilis.

Most medical students have more than enough knowledge to pass finals. Problems often arise in conveying that knowledge to the examiner in an organized manner. When asked a question either in the viva or as an essay question, spend a little while organizing your thoughts. In an essay you must write a plan. In a spoken answer make a swift plan in your head. The tips in this chapter are designed to help you make these plans.

There are certain key words which should elicit automatic responses; these responses act like a plan at the beginning of an essay. As an example, when asked

How would you make the *diagnosis* of carcinoma of the colon?

reply with the formula

The diagnosis of carcinoma of the colon is made by taking a history, examining the patient and carrying out investigations.

Then carry on to explain the diagnostic features of the history, the possible findings on examination and the diagnostic investigations, thereby avoiding the classic error of answering 'Barium enema' and forgetting that rectal bleeding and a change in bowel habit are the first clues in the diagnostic process.

There are a number of these key words which should elicit automatic responses which you must rehearse and memorize.

Discuss the *management* of haematemesis.

The management of haematemesis consists of making the diagnosis (by taking a history, examining the patient and carrying out investigations) and treating the patient.

What is the *treatment* for ingrowing toenails?

The treatment for ingrowing toenails may be conservative or operative.

It is very easy to forget in a surgical exam that the initial treatment, and often that most commonly employed, is conservative, involving advice on how to cut the nail and correct the deformity. Do not immediately offer ablation of the nail bed as the answer.

When asked about the *treatment* of a malignant condition remember that not only may the treatment be conservative or surgical, but the aim of treatment has to be established. Is it curative or palliative? If curative, then you may employ operative treatment, radiotherapy or chemotherapy. Remember also adjuvant radiotherapy, chemotherapy and hormonal treatment. If palliation is the aim then operation, radiotherapy, chemotherapy, hormonal therapy and immunotherapy may be employed. Finally, remember palliative care, the control of pain, psychological and emotional support for the patient and family and the role of the hospice.

What are the *complications* of haemorrhoidectomy?

The complications of haemorrhoidectomy are those of any surgical operation and those specifically associated with haemorrhoidectomy. These complications may be early, intermediate or late.

This avoids the pitfall of forgetting that the commonest complication of the operation is probably chest infection.

Any wider-ranging *discussion* of a disease should be considered under the headings of pathology, diagnosis and treatment. In a viva, this question may be phrased 'Tell me what you know about...' The same approach makes an excellent essay plan for those of you who still have to write them. The pathology forms a good introduction and should be dealt with according to the time-honoured mnemonic

In

A

Surgeon's

Gown

Physicians

May

Make

Some

Progress

reminding you of the headings

Incidence

Age,

Sex,

Geographical distribution

Predisposing factors

Macroscopic appearance

Microscopic appearance

Spread (for malignant disease)

Prognosis according to stage (for malignant disease)

Then proceed to a discussion of diagnosis and treatment as explained above.

The other general question which may appear in many guises both in the vivas and in the written papers concerns the *presentation* of malignant disease. This should be answered by referring to the history of the primary lesion, the history of possible secondaries and the history of non-specific features of the malignancy. Then turn to the physical signs of the primary tumour and the physical signs generated by the metastases. Finally, discuss the investigation of the primary tumour (definitive investigations) and the investigation of metastases (staging).

Finally, fluency in your examination of the short cases, in your presentation of the long case and in your answers in the viva create an impression of competence. There are three important ways to cultivate this fluency.

1. First, and most importantly, *see lots of patients*, take lots of histories and examine lots of long and short cases. Book learning, though important, cannot hide a lack of familiarity and contact with real patients.
2. Second, *practise exam technique*. Present histories and answer viva questions in exam conditions.

Do this with a colleague or even on your own. Practise spending a few seconds collecting your thoughts and making plans, as explained above. The answer, aiming to keep talking for the whole of the viva. If you keep talking, then what you say is likely to be right; when you stop the examiner will ask you another question – and this one you may not be able to answer.

3. Lastly, in the exam itself, after seeing your long case, in the few minutes you have *prepare your presentation to yourself* as you will recite it to the examiner, if possible without referring to your notes. Then ask yourself what questions the examiner is likely to ask and prepare the answers. You will usually be asked what you think the diagnosis or the differential diagnosis is and what investigations you would wish to order. You may then be asked about treatment.

We should at this stage wish you good luck with your surgical finals. However, after all the work you have done and after reading this book and following the advice in it and in this chapter, you really shouldn't need it. Good luck, anyway.

INDEX

INDEX